# Change Your Diet, Change Your Life

## 2019 Report

A Special Report
published by the editors of
*Tufts Health & Nutrition Letter*
in cooperation with
The Friedman School of Nutrition Science and Policy
at Tufts University

*Change Your Diet, Change Your Life*

Consulting Editor: Nicola McKeown, PhD, Scientist I, Jean Mayer USDA Human Nutrition Research Center on Aging at Tufts University and Associate Professor at the Friedman School of Nutrition Science and Policy at Tufts University

Author: Marsha McCulloch, MS, RDN
Update Author: Carrie Dennett, MPH, RDN
Creative Director, Belvoir Media Group: Judi Crouse
Editor, Belvoir Media Group: Cindy Foley
Production: Mary Francis McGavic

Publisher, Belvoir Media Group: Timothy H. Cole
Executive Editor, Book Division, Belvoir Media Group: Lynn Russo Whylly

ISBN 978-1-879620-95-7

To order additional copies of this report or for customer service questions, please call 877-300-0253, or write to Health Special Reports, 535 Connecticut Avenue, Norwalk, CT 06854-1713.

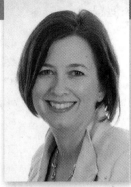

**Nicola McKeown, PhD**
Scientist at the Jean Mayer USDA Human Nutrition Research Center on Aging at Tufts University; Associate Professor at the Friedman School of Nutrition Science and Policy at Tufts University

Are you ready to embrace a healthy lifestyle? This may be easier said than done! Take a minute or two to reflect on your current diet and lifestyle habits without self-judgment. Would you like to make changes? Maybe you have some goals for improving your diet and/or lifestyle, but you're not sure of how to get started. Our 2019 edition of *Change Your Diet, Change Your Life* from the Friedman School of Nutrition Science and Policy at Tufts University will help put those lifestyle changes into motion, so you can live a better, more enjoyable life.

If this is your first year reading this report, welcome! If you are a returning reader, I hope that you'll be empowered to continue making small shifts toward incorporating heathier options into your eating plan. Adopting a healthy eating plan that tastes delicious and feels doable over the long term can be a powerful tool for helping to prevent, delay, manage, or even reverse some chronic health conditions.

One challenge many of us face is how to maintain a healthy body weight. How much we eat is influenced by how food looks and smells, how tasty it is, how long we sit at the table, how much other people are eating, the size of the package or container, and how much we're served. There's a lot of stimuli that we have to manage every time we think of eating. Throughout *Change Your Diet, Change Your Life,* you will find strategies to help you make healthier choices while still enjoying the experience of dining out with friends and family or eating your favorite meal or dessert.

The science of nutrition is moving forward at a fast pace. Throughout this report, we highlight notable findings from recent studies on diet and health in our "Year in Nutrition" boxes. We've also included a week's worth of new menus and recipes to help you make easy, tasty meals at home more often.

Think of each day as a new slate to start eating healthy, and remember a small shift in food choices can translate into substantial health benefits. Don't eat enough fruits? Consider drinking a smoothie in the morning. Not an adventurous cook? Start with simple recipes that double your vegetable intake. Enjoy a sandwich for lunch? Ask yourself if it can be improved by replacing mayo with hummus spread or adding more salad-based foods to your repertoire. Maybe you can swap out your traditional lunch for salads twice a week.

Making changes to your diet does requires you to question your current diet and how it's working for you. In other words, you need to be mindful about actively trying to make your diet better.

Be adventurous and bold in your dietary choices and be kind to yourself if you slip up. Tomorrow is another day!
Sincerely,

Nicola McKeown, PhD

# TABLE OF CONTENTS

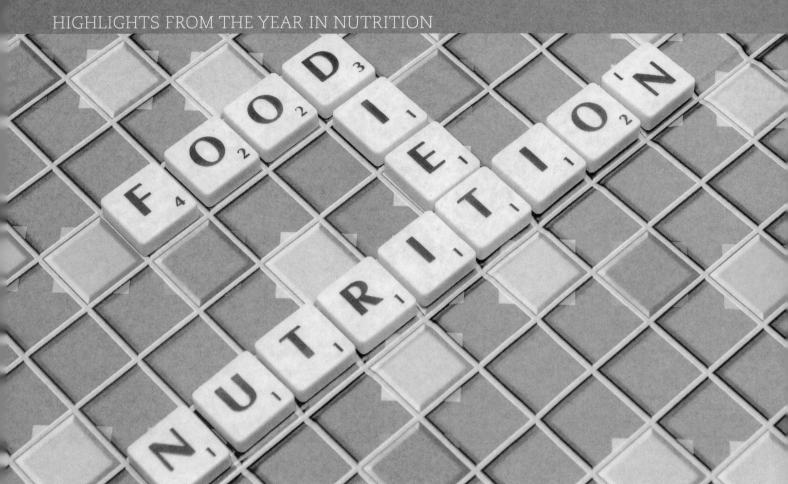

© Radub85 | Dreamstime

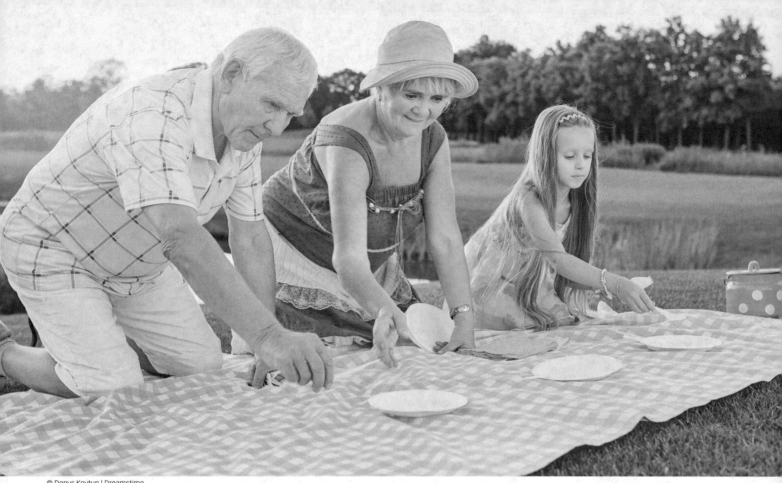

© Denys Kovtun | Dreamstime

Healthy eating and an active lifestyle can help you avoid a preventable, chronic health condition.

# 1 Invest in Your Health

Many things affect our health. A few, such as age and genetics, we can't control. However, lifestyle plays a major role, and we do have a say in that. Our diet—what we eat, not necessarily a weight-loss "diet"—along with stress, sleep, and physical activity, all affect how we feel today and how healthy we are tomorrow. When you eat well, stay active, manage stress, and get enough quality sleep, you increase your odds of staying strong and feeling your best for as long as possible. Let's start with food.

## Why Is Healthy Eating Important?

About half of all American adults have at least one preventable, chronic health condition, but *you* don't have to be one of them. Healthy eating is one of the most powerful tools for preventing chronic diseases such as cardiovascular disease and type 2 diabetes. The foods you choose can help you control your blood pressure and blood sugar, lower your total and "bad" (LDL) cholesterol, raise your "good" (HDL) cholesterol, lower your triglyceride levels, minimize cell damage, reduce systemic inflammation, and decrease your risk of heart attack, stroke, and certain kinds of cancer. If that's not enough, research shows that adults with healthier diets have better physical function, mental health, and general quality of life as they age.

What if you already have a chronic condition such as cardiovascular disease, diabetes, or kidney disease? The good news is that smart eating can help you manage or slow down the progression of these conditions. Recent research found that people at high genetic risk for coronary artery disease who met at least three out of four healthy lifestyle factors (no smoking, no obesity, regular physical activity, and a healthy diet) had a 46 percent lower risk of coronary events than high-risk individuals without healthy habits.

## Dietary Patterns

Nutrition science began as a search for ways to end malnutrition. Scientists wanted to understand which individual nutrients in what quantities were necessary for normal growth and health. While people still tend to focus on the effects of individual nutrients in the body ("vitamin C boosts the immune system," "calcium builds strong bones"), it has become clear that nutrients don't work alone—they work in synergy. In other words, the calcium in a glass of milk can't build strong bones effectively without the vitamin D, vitamin K, magnesium, and other nutrients from foods such as fish, fruits, and vegetables pitching in. This growing understanding has led to a shift in nutrition research and recommendations. Instead of focusing on individual vitamins, minerals, or food groups, the focus is on promoting healthier overall dietary patterns. We don't eat "nutrients," we eat foods—and we eat them combined into meals that, over time, make up our own dietary pattern.

A healthy eating pattern includes a variety of nutritious foods, such as vegetables, fruits, whole grains, legumes (beans, peas, and lentils), low-fat dairy, fish, poultry, lean meats, nuts, and seeds.

**THE YEAR IN NUTRITION**

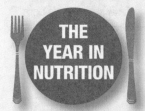

### For a Higher-Quality Diet, Give Up Grazing

Snacking is on the rise and not just between meals. More people are "grazing" on small amounts of food throughout the day rather than eating regular meals. While this may seem like a convenient way to keep hunger at bay and stay fueled, especially when busy, recent research suggests that grazing may lead to lower diet quality and sometimes higher body weight.

Using data from 4,544 adult participants in the Australian National Nutrition and Physical Activity Survey, the researchers compared a grazing eating pattern to conventional eating, (eating at typical meal times) and late-lunch patterns.

They found that a grazing dietary pattern resulted in lower dietary quality. The authors attribute this, in part, to the fact that vegetable intake was lower and intake of "discretionary foods" was higher compared to the other two patterns. These discretionary foods include sugary drinks, cookies, cakes, pastries, and processed meats. Grazers were also more likely to start eating later in the day and continue eating past 8 p.m. This appeared to have a modest but statistically significant effect on weight in women, as female grazers, on average, were more likely to have a body mass index (BMI) in the overweight or obese ranges and were specifically more likely to have central, or abdominal, obesity.

*American Journal of Clinical Nutrition,* October 2017

## Actual Eating Habits vs. Recommendations

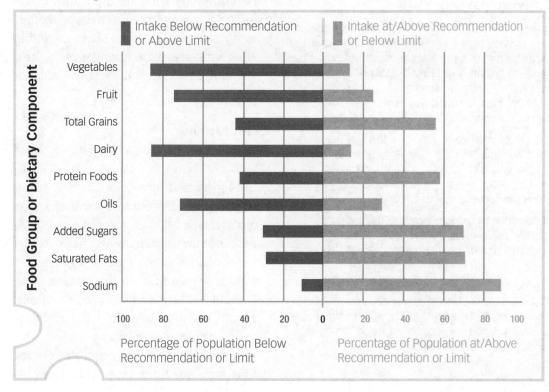

This graph shows the percentage of the U.S. population who are below or above each dietary recommendation or limit. The center line represents the recommended amount or limit. The consequences of falling above or below the center line depend on the food group or dietary component. For example, if you exceed the recommendation for servings of fruits or vegetables, particularly non-starchy ones, it could be beneficial (assuming you don't exceed your calorie needs). However, if you go beyond the limit for added sugars, saturated fats, and sodium, it could be harmful to your health.

Chart adapted from health.gov/dietaryguidelines/2015/guidelines

Unfortunately, actual eating habits usually don't match recommendations, and the eating pattern followed by about three-fourths of the U.S. population is low in vegetables, fruits, and dairy products.

There is more than one way to achieve a healthy eating pattern that incorporates the nutritious foods mentioned above. Your ideal dietary pattern can take into account your preferences, lifestyle, environment, and specific health needs, empowering you to make the changes and choices that work in your life. If you're concerned that healthful choices won't appeal to you, rest assured that you can retrain your palate and expand your dietary variety through repeated exposure to new foods. For example, research has found that people who were unfamiliar with pulses (beans, lentils, and peas) rated them more favorably after eating them for six weeks. In Chapter 2, you will be introduced to four dietary patterns—MyPlate, DASH, Mediterranean-style eating, and a plant-based diet—that have been shown to promote good health and help you age well.

## A Healthy Lifestyle

Eating well is a key element of a healthy lifestyle, but no health advice would be complete without mentioning the importance of physical activity and other facets of a healthy lifestyle, such as getting adequate sleep, reducing stress, and avoiding smoking and excessive alcohol consumption.

### Get Moving

Compared with less active people, those who are more physically active tend to live longer and have lower risks of many chronic diseases, such as cardiovascular disease, type 2 diabetes, obesity, and some cancers. Physical activity also helps reduce depression and slow down age-related muscle loss and cognitive decline. The *Physical Activity Guidelines for Americans*, established in 2008, offer sound guidance for planning your own physical activity routine, including how often to exercise and how to determine your exercise

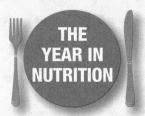

### Keeping Blood Vessels Healthy With Age

Blood pressure and stiffness of the artery walls both increase with age, raising the risk of developing cardiovascular disease. The good news is that it appears that age-related changes to blood vessels may be due to lifestyle more than age itself.

A review of research on factors that may affect vascular—or blood vessel—health found that moderate-intensity aerobic exercise appears to contribute to healthy vascular aging in adults who don't yet have high blood pressure. The authors also found that taking steps to reach a healthy weight by reducing calories—ideally in combination with a healthy eating plan and aerobic exercise—can reduce arterial stiffness and lower blood pressure.

The DASH (Dietary Approaches to Stop Hypertension) and Mediterranean dietary patterns are two good examples of how to eat for vascular health, in part because they are lower in sodium and higher in fruits and vegetables. These diets are also rich in flavonoids—a phytochemical found in citrus fruit, seeds, olive oil, tea, and red wine—which may contribute to lowering blood pressure.

The bottom line is that eating a healthy diet rich in fruits and vegetables, and exercising regularly, can matter more than age when it comes to preventing so-called "age-related" health conditions.

*Hypertension,* March 2018

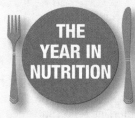

### Is Exercise the Best Prescription for Healthy Aging?

Many people find it harder to walk and easier to lose their balance as they age, but these changes aren't an inevitable part of aging. Not staying active can make it harder to be active, resulting in a loss of strength, mobility, and physical independence. The good news is that increasing physical activity by less than an hour a week could shift the tide in favor of better health and greater independence.

For The Lifestyle Interventions and Independence for Elders (LIFE) study, researchers randomly assigned 1,635 men and women ages 70 to 89 to either a physical activity program or a health education class for two years. All of the participants were physically inactive at the start of the study—getting less than 20 minutes of regular physical activity per week—and already had some functional limitations.

The physical activity group participated in twice-weekly classes that included walking, lower-body resistance exercises using ankle weights, a set of balance exercises, and a brief lower-body stretching routine. They also had personalized walking goals to meet outside of class.

The results? The more exercise people did, the better their physical function. The participants who added at least 43 minutes of physical activity each week—about the length of one of the LIFE physical activity classes—was enough to dramatically reduce the risk of physical disability. To stay strong, independent, and healthy, exercise is indeed good medicine, and it's never too late to start!

*PLOS ONE,* August 2018

## Physical Activity Guidelines

Each week, all adults should aim for:

☑ **Aerobic activity**

- Moderate-intensity
  150 minutes (2 hours and 30 minutes) aerobic activity in episodes of at least 10 minutes, and preferably, it should be spread throughout the week

  **OR**

- Vigorous-intensity
  75 minutes (1 hour and 15 minutes) of aerobic activity in episodes of at least 10 minutes, and preferably, it should be spread throughout the week

**PLUS**

☑ **Muscle-strengthening activities** that involve all major muscle groups two or more days a week.

**Tips:**

- If you cannot meet these guidelines, be as physically active as you are able.
- While vigorous activity "gets the job done" in less time, getting enough exercise of any intensity can improve health and longevity.
- For even more health benefits, increase aerobic activity to five hours a week of moderate intensity or 2½ hours of vigorous intensity.
- Older adults should do exercises that maintain or improve balance.
- If you have a chronic condition, learn whether and how your condition affects your ability to do regular physical activity safely.

## Determining Exercise Intensity

Although exercise intensity varies by individual, this chart gives you a general idea of what is commonly considered moderate- versus vigorous-intensity aerobic activity. In general, if you can carry on a conversation during exercise but need to stop speaking here or there, it is moderate-intensity activity. If you can only talk in short sentences, it's vigorous activity. If you can talk without any difficulty whatsoever, it's low intensity and you can likely pick up your pace.

© Bialasiewicz | Dreamstime

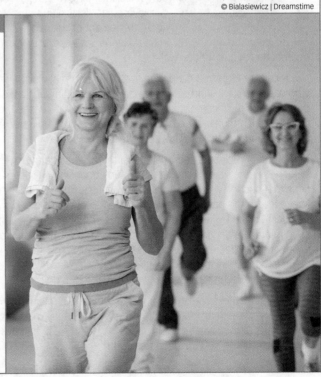

| MODERATE INTENSITY | VIGOROUS INTENSITY |
|---|---|
| • Ballroom or square dancing | • Backpacking |
| • Baseball or softball | • Cross-country skiing |
| • Bicycling less than 10 mph | • Ice hockey |
| • Bowling | • Ice skating |
| • Fishing and hunting | • Jogging or running |
| • Golf (without cart) | • Karate |
| • Juggling | • Kickboxing |
| • Kayaking | • Mountain biking |
| • Mopping or vacuuming | • Racquetball |
| • Mowing (power mower) | • Rock or mountain climbing |
| • Operating snow blower | • Rollerblading |
| • Shooting baskets | • Rowing |
| • Shuffleboard | • Shoveling snow |
| • Sweeping outside (garage, sidewalks) | • Soccer |
| • Tai chi | • Step aerobics (with 6- to 12-inch step) |
| • Tennis (doubles) | • Swimming laps |
| • Walking briskly on a level surface | • Tennis (singles) |
| • Water aerobics | • Volleyball, competitive |
| • Wii Fit Super Hula Hoop | • Water (aqua) jogging |

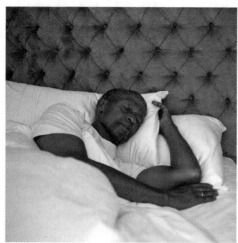
© Wavebreakmediamicro | Dreamstime

*A healthy night's sleep is just as important as diet and exercise.*

intensity. The good news is that recent research suggests that total duration of physical activity, rather than intensity, is most important to overall health and longevity, so choose activities that feel good to you and get moving!

## Get Your ZZZs

If you have trouble sleeping, you're not alone: An estimated 50 to 70 million American adults have a sleep or wakefulness disorder. The average person needs seven to eight hours of sleep per night. However, a study by the Centers for Disease Control and Prevention (CDC) found that more than a third of U.S. adults report getting less than seven hours of sleep per night. Research has shown that adequate sleep contributes to healthier blood pressure, cholesterol, and triglyceride levels. In a large observational study, scientists found that averaging more than seven hours of sleep per night was associated with a 22 percent lower risk of cardiovascular disease and a 43 percent lower risk of dying of cardiovascular causes, regardless of other lifestyle factors. These benefits were amplified when people also ate healthfully, exercised, limited alcohol intake, and avoided smoking. More recently, an observational study in 15,845 Swedish middle-aged to older adults observed that weight gain was linked to greater sleep problems. One potential explanation is that sleep impacts the hormones that signal whether you're hungry or full, so getting inadequate sleep may lead to increased hunger and higher calorie intake, including intake of added sugars.

## Stress Less

Chronic stress can lead to anxiety, insomnia, muscle pain, high blood pressure, and a weakened immune system. It also contributes to the development of heart disease and depression and is a factor in developing obesity. According to the American Psychological Association, 27 percent of adults say they eat to manage stress. While some people try to manage stress by turning to substances or behaviors that ultimately aren't good for health, there are ways to reduce stress in a healthy way.

## Making Changes

Adopting new behaviors is challenging for most people. One strategy for successful change involves the following steps:

- Identify areas for improvement in your lifestyle and share your goals for changing with a close friend or family member
- Pick one or two doable changes at a time
- Don't expect perfection and take each day as a new day

It's common to want to make big, sweeping changes when you decide to swap old habits for new, healthier ones, but small steps add up and make it easier to form habits that truly stick. Research has found that

---

**THE YEAR IN NUTRITION**

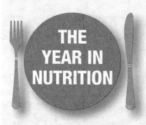
THE YEAR IN NUTRITION

### Sleeping More May Help Reduce Sugar Intake

Skimping on sleep—whether quantity or quality—is associated with a number of unwanted health outcomes, including weight gain and increased risk of cardiovascular disease and type 2 diabetes. Currently, about 37 percent of U.S. adults report sleeping 6 hours or less, even though the recommendations are to get 7 to 9 hours of sleep for optimal health and mental well-being.

In a recent randomized controlled study of 42 normal weight healthy adults who were habitual short sleepers—defined as getting at least 5 hours but less than 7 hours of sleep per night—participants who increased their sleep slightly consumed less sugar. Excess sugar intake is considered a risk factor for a number of health conditions, including cardiovascular disease.

Half of the participants kept their usual sleep schedule during the 4 weeks of the study, while the other half were educated about sleep hygiene—habits and practices that support a good night's sleep. These include avoiding excessive caffeine intake late in the day and not going to bed too full or too hungry. The participants practicing sleep hygiene spent an average of 55 minutes more in bed, resulting in an average of 21 additional minutes of actual sleep. Interestingly, although they experienced a decrease in sleep quality, possibly because they weren't used to being in bed longer, the sleep hygiene group significantly reduced their intake of added sugars, even though they were not asked to do so.

These pilot results suggest that if you fall shy of the minimum 7 hours of recommended sleep, getting even a little bit more sleep may make it easier to moderate your intake of the sweet stuff. Try practicing good sleep habits and practices to try to gain another ½ hour of sleep per night!

*American Journal of Clinical Nutrition,* January 2018

it can take anywhere from 18 to 254 days for a new habit to become a comfortable norm. The good news is, this same research shows that slipping up now and then doesn't affect the habit-forming process. If you notice you've fallen off track, simply start again and repeat as often as necessary. Research suggests that more than 45 percent of our eating activities are based on habits, so once you build new habits, the healthier choice will become the more automatic choice. Think progress, not perfection.

While the impact of dietary choices on health and quality of life can be dramatic, the changes you make to your diet don't have to be. For example, research presented at the 2017 scientific sessions of the American Heart Association reported that simply eating more fruits and vegetables could significantly reduce the incidence of disability and premature death from heart disease.

Making small, positive changes in the way you eat will help you create a healthy eating pattern that makes sense for you. For example, have some raw veggies with a little hummus as a late-afternoon snack instead of cheese and crackers and make a goal to eat at least one fish meal a week (two is optimal) if fish isn't in your usual repertoire. Watch for "Smart Shift" boxes in the margins of each chapter in this report for simple changes that will add up to a healthier overall dietary pattern.

A healthy dietary pattern can open the door to a world of better health and preserve or improve your quality of life. With reasonable goals, self-compassion, and a willingness to start again if you find yourself faltering, you can change your diet and your life. Invest in your health—you're worth it. This report hopefully will serve as a foundation to help you get started, or continue, on your journey.

## Managing Stress

When untreated, chronic stress can result in serious health conditions and contribute to the development of serious health problems, such as heart disease and depression, as well as weight gain. According to the American Psychological Association, research recommends the following techniques to help handle stress:

- **Take a break from the stressor:** Give yourself permission to step away from the source of your stress. Even just 20 minutes of self-care helps, such as a bath, a walk, listening to music, or some meditation, for example.

- **Exercise:** Exercise benefits your mind as well as your body. A regular exercise routine is ideal, but even a 20-minute walk, run, swim, or dance session in the midst of a stressful time can give an immediate effect that can last for several hours.

- **Smile and laugh:** Our brains are interconnected with our emotions and facial expressions. Laughing and smiling can help relieve tension.

- **Get social support:** Sharing your concerns or feelings with someone you trust can help relieve stress.

- **Meditate:** Research has shown that even meditating briefly can reap immediate benefits. Meditation can help the mind and body relax and focus.

- **Pursue a hobby:** Gardening, playing music, creating art, bird-watching, or anything else that brings you joy is a great way to manage stress.

## DIETLIFE TIPS

### Small Steps to Healthy Habits

The key to moving toward health-promoting behaviors is to make gradual changes to your habits. The following tips may help.

☑ **Make sure you have a real desire to change.** Weigh the pros and cons of the change you're considering. Keep in mind that it's normal to feel some ambivalence about changing—it can help to research the benefits of the change you're considering if you need more "pros" for your list!

☑ **Start with a small change that feels manageable.** Succeeding at that tiny change will boost your confidence and inspire you to keep going.

☑ **Identify cues.** Habitual behaviors are often triggered by specific links to other actions (e.g., "I'm done with dinner, so it must be time for dessert"). Identifying your cues allows you to change your response (e.g., "I'm done with dinner, so it's time to take a nice evening stroll"). The goal is to learn to respond thoughtfully, rather than react mindlessly.

☑ **Change your environment, if necessary.** Willpower will only take you so far. If you can't resist tempting treats, keep them out of the house and make healthier options easily available. If you always hit the donut shop on your way to work, change your route so you don't pass it.

☑ **Celebrate progress.** No matter how small your new healthy behavior is, take time to feel proud. Patting yourself on the back fires off positive emotions that reinforce the new behavior.

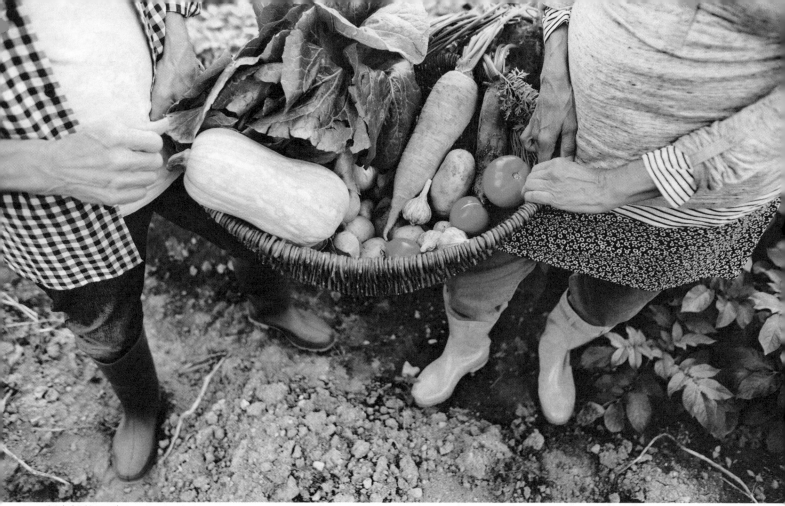

Every healthy eating pattern includes vegetables, which are even more satisfying when you grow them yourself.

## 2 Dietary Patterns

No single food, meal, or even day of eating makes or breaks our path to better nutrition and health. What matters most is what and how much you eat over time. In other words, your overall "dietary pattern." Your dietary pattern reflects the quantity, proportion, variety of different foods and drinks in your diet, and the frequency and combination with which they are habitually consumed. Of course, not all dietary patterns are created equal, and the dietary pattern followed by many people in this country—the "typical American diet" or "Western dietary pattern"—gets low marks with respect to its nutrient composition. Why? Because this dietary pattern is high in processed red meat, refined grains, and sugary foods and beverages. Consequently, it is also high in saturated fats and sodium and low in many nutrients. It is not a diet that promotes health and well-being.

Is there one perfect eating pattern? No … even though humans are amazingly similar—we share more than 99 percent of our DNA—we don't all respond to food in the same way. For example, some people thrive with fewer carbohydrate-rich foods, while others do best with less dietary fat. So, it's important that you recognize what's right for you may not be right for someone else.

### Healthy Eating Habits Protect Against Temptation

We often think that people should use self-control and willpower to make choices that support long-term health goals instead of immediate gratification, but that's easier said than done.

Our eating habits are strongly tied to context cues, such as time of day and physical location. A classic study offered participants stale popcorn while they watched a movie. People who usually ate popcorn at the movies ate significant amounts of the stale popcorn. When the same people were offered stale popcorn when watching a music video, however, they did not eat it. Movies were such a strong cue to eat popcorn that they ate it even though they admitted it tasted bad! It's estimated that more than 45 percent of eating choices may be habitual—so not really choices at all. If we form habits of consuming smaller portions of food and choosing healthier options, we're more likely to do so even when tempted to do otherwise.

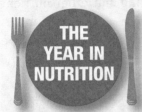

THE YEAR IN NUTRITION

DIETLIFE TIPS

### Yes, a Better Diet Is Linked to Better Health

Researchers recently looked at the link between diet quality and risk of developing chronic diseases. The study examined how following a diet that meets the criteria of the Healthy Eating Index (HEI), the Alternative Healthy Eating Index (AHEI), or the DASH (Dietary Approaches to Stop Hypertension) eating plan impacts health. The HEI includes foods that correspond to the current *Dietary Guidelines for Americans,* while the AHEI considers a few additional factors that the HEI doesn't, including alcohol use, vitamin use, white-to-red meat ratio, and polyunsaturated-to-saturated fat ratio.

Based on a meta-analysis of data from prospective cohort studies (data from 68 reports, including more than 1.6 million participants), the authors found that the highest quality diets, as measured by HEI, AHEI, or DASH, were associated with not just reduced risk of death from all causes, but specifically with lower rates of cardiovascular disease, type 2 diabetes, cancer, and neurodegenerative disease like Alzheimer's or Parkinson's disease. The AHEI appeared to offer the greatest protection against neurodegenerative diseases.

Looking more closely at cancer risk, the study found that the greatest reductions were for colorectal, esophageal, lung, gallbladder, pancreatic, prostate, head and neck, and liver cancer. Among cancer survivors, a diet that closely mirrors the HEI was associated with reduced risk of death from cancer or other causes in women.

While the data used in this study was observational and, therefore can't show cause-and-effect, the findings are still promising and consistent with the message that better diet quality is one modifiable risk factor that can protect our health.

*Journal of the Academy of Nutrition and Dietetics,* January 2018

- ▶ **Think big picture.** How does your overall dietary pattern look? Is it rich in healthy foods?
- ▶ **Customize.** There is no single perfect diet. A healthful dietary pattern can be adapted to meet your individual needs and tastes.
- ▶ **Pick a pattern.** MyPlate, the DASH diet, and a Mediterranean-style diet are all research-based dietary patterns that support good health.
- ▶ **Go more plant-based.** A healthful diet is rich in plant foods such as fruits, vegetables, whole grains, legumes, nuts, and seeds.
- ▶ **Be mindful of portion size.** No matter how healthy your food choices, how much you eat matters.

You may need to tweak a specific dietary pattern to make it healthier for you. A 2017 study that was part of the larger Nurses' Health Study found that what's important for reducing health risks isn't so much which healthy eating pattern participants chose, just that they stuck to it.

While healthy eating patterns have some foods in common—vegetables, fruits, whole grains, nuts, and legumes—there is a lot of flexibility to tailor them to fit your tastes based on budget, time, cooking skills, culture, and traditions.

In this chapter, we'll discuss four dietary patterns that multiple studies shows contribute to better health: MyPlate, the Mediterranean diet, the DASH diet, and plant-based diets.

## The MyPlate Method

Every five years, the federal government updates the *Dietary Guidelines for Americans* (DGA) to offer the latest science-based advice on eating for good health. Using the DGA as a foundation, the U.S. Department of Agriculture (USDA) developed MyPlate as a simple visual guide to illustrate a healthful eating pattern. The website, ChooseMyPlate.gov, is full of tips and tools to help you make better food choices that align with your personal dietary preferences.

The MyPlate icon depicts four food groups that should be included in every meal: fruits and vegetables, grains, protein, and dairy.

### USDA-Recommended Food Patterns

The USDA Food Patterns lists daily amounts of foods to eat from the five major food groups based on an individual's calorie needs, consistent with MyPlate recommendations. Below are examples of eating patterns recommended for those who need 1,600 calories (typical for sedentary women age 51 and older) or 2,000 calories (typical for sedentary men age 51 and older) daily.

| Daily Amount of Food from Each Group | 1,600-CALORIE DIET | 2,200-CALORIE DIET |
|---|---|---|
| Fruits | 1½ cups | 2 cups |
| Vegetables | 2 cups | 2½ cups |
| Grains | 5 oz-eq | 6 oz-eq |
| Proteins | 5 oz-eq | 5½ oz-eq |
| Dairy | 3 cups | 3 cups |
| Oils* | 22 g | 27 g |
| Calorie limit for solid fats and added sugars | 121 | 28 |

Note: g = grams; oz-eq = ounce equivalents, which are described in the chapters covering each food group.
*Approximately 5 to 6½ teaspoons

**USDA MyPlate**

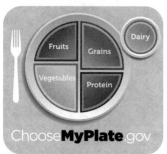

- ▶ **Fruits and vegetables should make up half of your plate.** Choose a variety of colors and types (see Chapter 3 for more on fruits and vegetables).
- ▶ **Grains should make up one-quarter of your plate.** Try to make at least half the grains you eat whole grains, such as whole-wheat bread, oatmeal, brown rice, and whole-grain pasta. To make meals more interesting and get a wider variety of nutrients, consider less traditional choices, such as barley, quinoa, bulgur, amaranth, and wheat berries (see Chapter 4 for more on whole grains).
- ▶ **Protein-rich foods should make up the remaining one-quarter of your plate.** These include foods such as fish, lean meat, chicken, eggs, tofu, beans, nuts, and nut butters. (See Chapter 5 for more on protein.)
- ▶ **Dairy foods,** which are also protein-rich, include items such as milk, yogurt, and cottage cheese. (See Chapters 5 and 8 for more on dairy.)

## Tufts' MyPlate for Older Adults

Although most nutritional guidance is "ageless," you can make some adjustments to your eating pattern that will help you meet the changing needs of your body as you age. Calorie requirements tend to decrease with aging, but other nutrient needs increase with age, so it is important to make every bite count. If you are concerned that you may be low in some nutrients, talk to your doctor.

To address the special concerns of older Americans, nutrition scientists at Tufts' Human Nutrition Research Center on Aging (HNRCA) created "MyPlate for Older Adults" (hnrca.tufts.edu/myplate).

## A Mediterranean-Style Diet

In general, a Mediterranean-style diet is rich in fruits, vegetables, whole grains, beans, nuts, and olive oil, and features fish and seafood but little red meat. Several health benefits have been attributed to following this dietary pattern including improved cardiovascular health, reduced risk of metabolic syndrome (a cluster of health problems including high blood pressure, elevated blood sugar, abnormal blood cholesterol and triglycerides, and excess abdominal fat) and reduced risk of stroke. Recent research even suggests that following a Mediterranean-style eating plan may reduce the risk of frailty in older women with type 2 diabetes. Furthermore, it may protect against

| Nutrients of Concern for Older Adults | |
|---|---|
| **NUTRIENT OF CONCERN** | **TOP FOOD SOURCES** |
| Protein | Meat, poultry, fish/seafood, dairy products, soy foods, legumes, nuts, seeds, quinoa |
| Omega-3 fatty acids | Fatty fish (herring, salmon, sardines, trout), ground flaxseeds/flaxseed oil, walnuts/walnut oil, chia seeds, tofu (firm), eggs from hens fed omega-3s, canola oil, soybean oil |
| Fiber | Whole grains, legumes, fruits, vegetables, nuts, and seeds |
| Calcium | Dairy products, almonds, spinach and other dark leafy greens, soybeans; fortified foods including ready-to-eat cereals, orange juice, milk substitutes and tofu prepared with calcium sulfate |
| Magnesium | Brown rice, corn, and other whole grains, beans, almonds, dark leafy greens, seeds; fortified foods including many ready-to-eat cereals |
| Potassium | Beans, orange juice, potato/sweet potato, soybeans, canned tomato products, dried apricots, plantains, winter squash, cabbage, nuts, yogurt, broccoli, cantaloupe, bananas |
| Vitamin B₁₂ | Fish/shellfish, meat, dairy, eggs; many ready-to-eat cereals and nutritional yeast are fortified |
| Vitamin D | Fish/seafood (herring, salmon, mackerel, sardines, trout, oysters, shrimp), eggs, mushrooms (especially those exposed to ultraviolet light); fortified foods including milk, orange juice, and cereals (Vitamin D Is also made by the body during exposure to sunlight) |

age-related macular degeneration and dementia, two additional health conditions linked to aging.

It's never too late to switch to a Mediterranean diet. Oldways, a nonprofit food and nutrition education organization, in partnership with the Harvard School of Public Health and the World Health Organization, created a Mediterranean Diet Pyramid. For more information on moving toward a Mediterranean-style diet, visit the Oldways website at oldwayspt.org.

## DASH: Dietary Approaches to Stop Hypertension

According to the Centers for Disease Control and Prevention (CDC), nearly one in three American Adults have hypertension. If you're one of them, you may want to consider a hypertension diet in line with the Dietary Approaches to Stop Hypertension

(DASH) pattern—a pattern recognized to lower blood pressure.

DASH emphasizes limiting sodium to under 2,300 milligrams (mg) per day, in addition to focusing on eating plenty of foods rich in nutrients that help to lower blood pressure, including potassium, magnesium, and calcium. Recommendations include eating plenty of fruits, vegetables, and whole grains, consuming nuts, seeds, and legumes several times a week, keeping dairy products low-fat or fat-free and meats lean, and limiting fats, oils, sweets, and added sugars.

Research has found the DASH diet may help to lower stroke risk by reducing plaque buildup in the arteries. Additionally, DASH may help protect against other medical conditions, including osteoporosis, kidney stones, diabetes, and some cancers, and can slow the progression of both heart

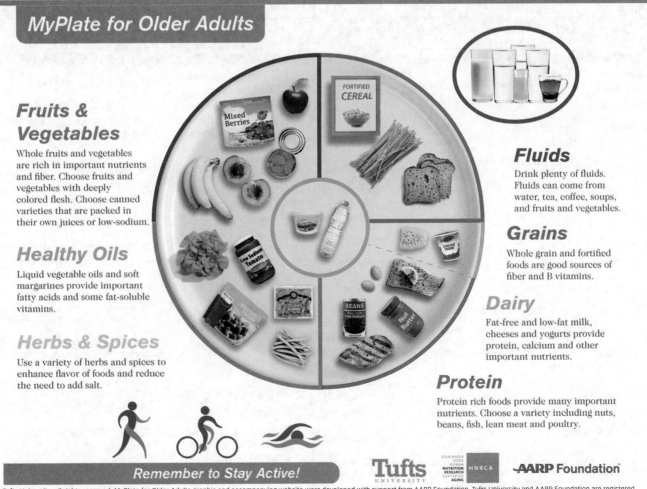

## MyPlate for Older Adults

### Fruits & Vegetables
Whole fruits and vegetables are rich in important nutrients and fiber. Choose fruits and vegetables with deeply colored flesh. Choose canned varieties that are packed in their own juices or low-sodium.

### Healthy Oils
Liquid vegetable oils and soft margarines provide important fatty acids and some fat-soluble vitamins.

### Herbs & Spices
Use a variety of herbs and spices to enhance flavor of foods and reduce the need to add salt.

### Fluids
Drink plenty of fluids. Fluids can come from water, tea, coffee, soups, and fruits and vegetables.

### Grains
Whole grain and fortified foods are good sources of fiber and B vitamins.

### Dairy
Fat-free and low-fat milk, cheeses and yogurts provide protein, calcium and other important nutrients.

### Protein
Protein rich foods provide many important nutrients. Choose a variety including nuts, beans, fish, lean meat and poultry.

**Remember to Stay Active!**

Tufts UNIVERSITY · JEAN MAYER USDA HUMAN NUTRITION RESEARCH CENTER ON AGING · HNRCA · AARP Foundation

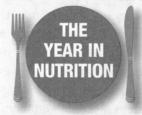

## Vegetarian and Mediterranean Diets Are Good for the Heart and Waistline

It used to be that nutrition research focused on specific nutrients or foods, but in the last decade or so, attention has turned to dietary patterns. Why? Because we don't eat nutrients or foods by themselves—we eat them in meals as part of overall patterns. Research has shown that certain dietary patterns may be effective for promoting a healthy weight and healthy heart. A recent study tackled this question: What's better for reducing weight and cardiovascular disease risk—a vegetarian or Mediterranean diet?

Turns out both may be great. In the study, 118 overweight omnivores with a low-to-moderate risk for developing cardiovascular disease were randomized to eat a low-calorie vegetarian diet or a low-calorie Mediterranean diet for three months. The only difference between the diets was that the Mediterranean diet included meat, poultry, and fish, while the vegetarian diet did not.

The two eating patterns proved equally effective at reducing body weight and body fat and lowering body mass index (BMI). However, the vegetarian diet did a better job at reducing LDL cholesterol levels, while the Mediterranean diet was superior for lowering triglyceride levels. Both of these largely plant-based diets met current dietary guidelines, which call for a varied, nutritious eating pattern rich in fruits, vegetables, legumes, whole grains, and nuts, while limiting excess calories and saturated fat. The good news is that this helps confirm that there's no one right way to eat, allowing you to find an eating pattern that suits your tastebuds and your health.

*Circulation, March 2018*

## Guide to the DASH Diet (Use this chart to help you plan your daily menus.)

| FOOD GROUP | CALORIES PER DAY* | | SAMPLE SERVING SIZES | | COMMENTS |
|---|---|---|---|---|---|
| | 1,600 | 2,000 | | | |
| Grains (mostly whole) | 6 servings | 6 to 8 servings | • 1 slice bread<br>• 1 oz dry cereal | • ½ cup cooked rice, pasta, or cereal | Provide energy and fiber |
| Vegetables | 3 to 4 | 4 to 5 | • 1 cup leafy greens<br>• ½ cup vegetable juice | • ½ cup cut-up raw or cooked vegetables | Provide potassium, magnesium, and fiber |
| Fruits | 4 | 4 to 5 | • 1 medium fruit<br>• ¼ cup dried fruit | • ½ cup fresh, frozen, or canned fruit<br>• ½ cup fruit juice | Provide potassium, magnesium, and fiber |
| Milk products (fat-free or low-fat) | 2 to 3 | 2 to 3 | • 1 cup milk or yogurt | • 1½ oz cheese | Provide calcium and protein |
| Lean meats, fish, poultry, and eggs | 3 to 4 or less | 6 or less | • 1 whole egg<br>• 2 egg whites | • 1 oz cooked lean meat, poultry, or fish | Provide protein and magnesium; limit egg yolks to 4 per week |
| Nuts, seeds, and legumes | 3 to 4 per week | 4 to 5 per week | • ⅓ cup (1½ oz) nuts<br>• 2 Tbsp nut butter | • 2 Tbsp (½ oz) seeds<br>• ½ cup cooked legumes (dried beans, peas) | Provide energy, magnesium, protein, and fiber |
| Fats and oils | 2 | 2 to 3 | • 1 tsp soft margarine<br>• 1 tsp olive oil<br>• 1 Tbsp mayonnaise | • 1 Tbsp regular salad dressing<br>• 2 Tbsp light salad dressing | Also choose lower-fat foods |
| Sweets and added sugars | 3 or less per week | 5 or less per week | • 1 Tbsp sugar<br>• 1 Tbsp jelly or jam | • ½ cup sorbet, gelatin<br>• 1 cup lemonade | Sweets should be low in fat |
| Sodium, maximum limit | 2,300 mg** | 2,300 mg** | • 1 tsp salt = 2,300 mg sodium | | Packaged foods are a major sodium source |

*Sedentary women age 51+ need around 1,600 calories per day; sedentary men age 51+ need around 2,000 calories per day.
**For individuals with prehypertension or hypertension, further sodium reduction to 1,500 mg per day can result in even greater blood pressure reduction.
Abbreviations: oz = ounce; Tbsp = tablespoon; tsp = teaspoon; mg = milligrams.
Source: *Dietary Guidelines for Americans, 2010* and *Dietary Guidelines for Americans, 2015-2020,* 8th ed.

and kidney diseases. (Note: If you already have chronic kidney disease, you should speak with your doctor and dietitian before starting any new diets, since you may have special restrictions. The DASH diet should not be used by people on dialysis.)

The DASH dietary pattern is not just for people with high blood pressure; it is a wise choice for anyone who is interested in protecting his or her health.

## A Plant-Based Diet

A plant-powered diet is a great choice for individuals who want to cut out animal products altogether, as well as those who just want to incorporate more healthful foods into their eating plan. A dietary pattern that emphasizes more plant foods and fewer animal foods may help reduce the risk of many common conditions, such as obesity, high blood pressure, heart disease, cancer, and diabetes, and it may also help you live longer. Plus, eating a variety of fruits and vegetables is good for increasing the diversity of your gut microbiota, which emerging research suggests is important for our health.

Many studies have linked plant-based diets to health benefits. For example, one research review of 96 different studies found that eating a lacto-ovo-vegetarian diet (a diet that includes eggs and dairy but no animal flesh) for four years or more was linked with a 25 percent reduced risk of ischemic heart disease and an 8 percent reduced risk of cancer. People who followed a vegan diet (a diet that contains no animal products) had a 15 percent reduced risk of cancer. Additionally, data showed that total cholesterol, LDL ("bad") cholesterol, blood sugar levels, and body mass index (BMI) were lower in vegetarians and vegans than in omnivores who eat both plant and animal foods, including meat. Other research found that vegans had a 16 percent lower risk of developing colorectal cancer over a seven-year period compared with non-vegetarians, while pescatarians (also spelled "pescetarian"), who eat fish

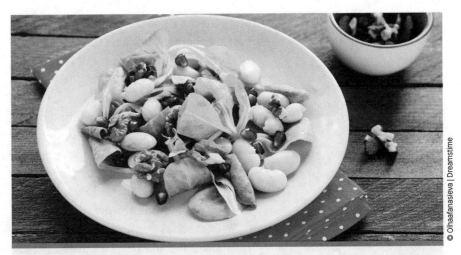

© Olhaafanasieva | Dreamstime

## Nutrients of Concern for Vegans

When not planned carefully, vegetarian and vegan diets can fall short on vitamin $B_{12}$, vitamin D, omega-3 fats, calcium, iodine, iron, and zinc, especially if eggs and dairy products are excluded. Here's where to find these important nutrients in plant-based sources, and recommendations for supplements, if needed.

### Vitamin $B_{12}$

- $B_{12}$-fortified non-dairy milks and meat substitutes
- $B_{12}$-fortified breakfast cereals and nutrition bars
- $B_{12}$-fortified nutritional yeast
- $B_{12}$ supplement (25 micrograms daily)

### Vitamin D

- Sun exposure
- Fortified foods
- Supplements (plant-based, such as from lichen), especially during winter months
- Vitamin D fortified mushrooms

### Calcium

- Green, leafy vegetables, especially bok choy, broccoli, collards, and kale
- Dried figs
- Almonds and almond butter
- Tahini (sesame seed butter)
- Calcium-fortified juices and non-dairy milks
- Tofu made with calcium sulfate or calcium chloride

### Iron*

- Cashews
- Beans
- Seeds, such as pumpkin
- Grains
- Dark-green vegetables, such as spinach
- Tofu and tempeh
- Dried fruits, such as raisins
- Iron-fortified foods
- Using iron cookware

### Zinc

- Soy products
- Legumes
- Nuts and seeds
- Whole grains
- Wheat germ
- Zinc-fortified foods, such as breakfast cereal

### Omega-3 fats (ALA, EPA, or DHA)

- Ground flaxseed
- Walnuts
- Canola and soybean oils
- Hemp-seed products
- Seaweed, such as kelp
- Algae-based marine supplements
- Non-dairy milks and cereal bars fortified with DHA (docosahexaenoic acid)

*Consume with vitamin C rich fruits and vegetables to boost iron absorption. Soaking and sprouting beans, seeds, and grains also improves iron absorption, as does leavening of bread.

and other seafood but no meat or poultry, had a 43 percent reduced risk.

Cutting out animal products removes a major source of protein in the Western diet (see Chapter 5 for more on protein). Fortunately, plant foods, including beans, lentils, nuts, and even some grains, can provide the protein you need. There are certain amino acids (the building blocks of proteins) that your body can't make, so they must come from food; these are called essential amino acids. Plant foods typically have smaller amounts of these essential amino acids than animal proteins, but it's not difficult to get enough if you eat a variety of plants. At one time, it was thought that people who excluded animal proteins had to combine plant foods (such as eating rice with beans) so that they would get all the essential amino acids at the same meal, but it's now known that eating a variety of plant-based foods over the course of a day— including legumes, nuts, seeds, and whole grains—is sufficient to provide you with the amino acids you need.

Soy is one of the few plant foods that contains all the essential amino acids.

Soybeans, edamame (immature soybeans), tofu, and tempeh are excellent protein choices, but soy-based "fake" meats, such as vegetarian burgers, hot dogs, and cold cuts, are highly processed and often are laden with salt, artificial colors and flavors, and other additives. Like soy, the grain quinoa also provides all the essential amino acids.

To experience the health benefits of a vegetarian diet, it's important to make healthful food choices overall and not simply avoid meat. Although potato chips, doughnuts, and soft drinks are technically plant foods, they're far from healthy. In fact, a 2017 study found that a plant-based diet that emphasizes less-healthy foods increases the risk of coronary heart disease, while a diet high in whole grains, fruits, vegetables, nuts, legumes, plant oils, and tea or coffee decreased risk by 25 percent. People who are vegetarians or vegans also need to be aware of potential nutritional deficiencies associated with diets that contain few or no animal foods. Plant-based eaters need to be particularly thoughtful about how they will get specific "nutrients of concern" from food or from supplements.

**SMART SHIFT**

### Ideas for Increasing Your Intake of Plant Foods

A dietary pattern that includes plenty of plant foods (fruits, vegetables, whole grains, beans, nuts, and seeds) is associated with better health. Here are some examples of how easy it can be to add plant foods:

- Keep ready-to-eat fruits and vegetables in visible, easy-to-grab places.
- Toss veggies into your morning eggs.
- Top whole-grain cereals with fresh or dried fruit, nuts, or seeds.
- Top oatmeal with fruit and nuts or cook it with grated apple or finely diced dates for natural sweetness and fiber.
- Choose whole-grain breads, pastas, and crackers.
- Load sandwiches with extra veggies.
- Use sliced fruit, such as bananas and apples, instead of jelly on peanut butter sandwiches.
- Toss extra veggies, beans, and whole grains into soups, stews, chili, and stir-fries.
- Make "kitchen sink" salads with greens, veggies, beans, proteins, nuts, seeds, fresh or dried fruits, and anything else that suits your fancy.
- Mix pasta half-and-half with cooked veggies for a hearty pasta primavera.
- Try eating meatless meals one day a week.
- Reach for fruit as a healthy sweet.
- Instead of rice or potatoes, experiment with the wide variety of whole grains available on supermarket shelves; try quinoa, buckwheat, millet, farro, wheat berries, freekeh, and other options.

## Portion Control

Even when you're making healthy food choices, the size of your food portions matter with respect to your daily caloric intake. However, being thin doesn't necessarily translate to better health, so don't choose a dietary pattern simply because you think it might promote weight loss. It's the diet quality that matters. That said, being overweight can have an impact on health (see the section on obesity in Chapter 9). Eating oversized portions can lead to weight gain because—whether they're healthy or not—all foods and most beverages have calories. When foods are "energy-dense"—providing a lot of calories, without much volume from fiber and water—it's easy to consume excess calories. Eating a daily salad composed of leafy greens and other non-starchy vegetables is a great strategy to fill you up without going overboard on calories because it's rich in nutrients, water, and fiber without being energy-dense.

Managing portion sizes in today's food environment is a constant challenge. How much we eat is influenced by how food looks and smells, how tasty it is, how long we sit at the table, how much other people are eating, the size of the package or container, and how much we're served. A review of 72 controlled trials on portion control found that people eat and drink more when they are offered larger-sized portions, packages, or plates than when offered smaller-sized versions of the same food or meal. This is a big concern for all of us when we consider that restaurant portions and package sizes have increased substantially over the past few decades. A typical muffin in the United States, for example, is more than three times bigger than the standard USDA serving size, and a serving of pasta offered at your favorite restaurant could be up to five times as large. Being mindful of the size of the plate or the serving size is important because, as we become accustomed to seeing these portions, we may see them as the norm rather than the exception. See Chapter 9 for tips on managing portion sizes.

## Putting it All Together

All three of the research-driven dietary patterns discussed above—MyPlate, DASH, and the Mediterranean-style diet—are very similar. Notably, they all contain more plant foods and less red meat than the typical Western diet. As you will see in the following chapters, there's no doubt that these choices are good for your health. Use the dietary pattern that best fits your lifestyle as a guide and fill it in with specific food choices and meals that appeal to you. Use the MyPlate image as a guide to manage portion size and proportion. Be sure when you add healthful foods to your diet that they're replacing less healthful choices rather than being added on top of them. Remember that each positive change you make is a shift in the right direction.

### Comparing Dietary Patterns

The basic framework for all the dietary patterns discussed in this chapter is very similar! This chart shows how much they have in common.

| DIETARY PATTERN | UNIQUE | SIMILAR | THE SAME |
|---|---|---|---|
| DGA/MyPlate | • Translated into MyPlate visual tool to simplify meeting intake goals | • Recommend low-fat and nonfat dairy<br>• Suggest moderate amounts of lean meat/fish/poultry | • Research shows numerous health benefits<br>• Emphasis on fruits, vegetables, and whole grains<br>• Include legumes (beans, lentils, peas), nuts, and seeds<br>• Provide heart-healthy fats |
| DASH | • Emphasis on limiting sodium intake (less than 2,300 mg/day) | | |
| Mediterranean | • Emphasis on olive oil as source of fats<br>• Specifically recommends red wine | | |
| Plant-based | • Emphasis on plant-based foods | • Can be vegan, vegetarian, or include fish/seafood and limited meat/poultry | |

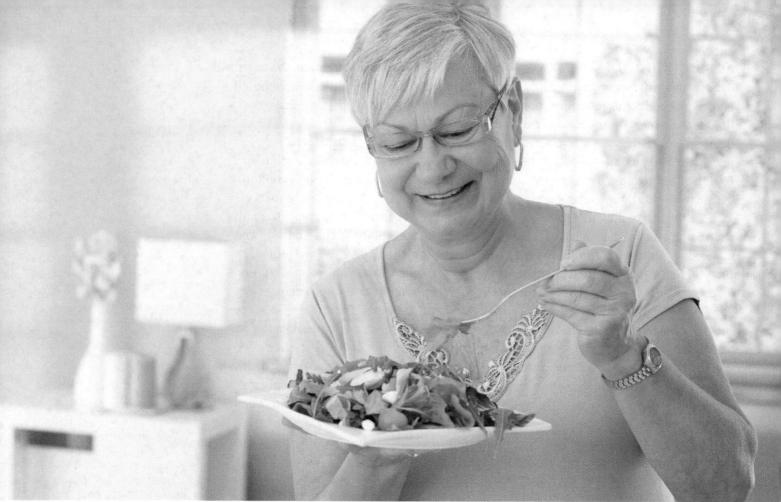

A leafy green salad can help fill you up and prevent cognitive decline as you age.

# 3 Fruits and Vegetables

Fruit is nature's perfect sweet, and vegetables are the common denominator in any healthy eating pattern. Whether you reach for a piece of juicy summer fruit, a crisp green salad, or a savory stir-fry, not only are you delighting your taste buds, you are making better food choices that will positively impact your health. You would be hard-pressed to find a health condition that a diet rich in fruits and vegetables doesn't play a role in preventing. Cancer, heart disease, stroke, and type 2 diabetes are a few of the major conditions that can be avoided with increased intakes of fruits and vegetables. A leafy green salad a day could even help prevent age-related cognitive decline. Eating lots of fruits and veggies in general may even help you live longer—allowing you ample time to enjoy more of that sweet summer fruit.

## Recommendations

Adults should aim to eat at least 2 to 3 cups of vegetables and 1½ to 2 cups of fruit daily. A report from the CDC showed that only 13 percent of people surveyed met the fruit recommendation and fewer than 9 percent of people ate the recommended amount of vegetables. How can you beat those numbers? Start by eating a fruit, a vegetable, or both at each meal and snack. It may help to brush up on what counts as a cup of vegetables or a cup of fruit.

There's good reason to pile on the fruits and veggies. A meta-analysis of 95 studies that included information from about

## DIETLIFE TIPS

- **Aim for a fruit and/or veggie at every meal and snack.** Choosing at least one serving of produce every time you eat goes a long way toward getting the recommended amount of fruits and vegetables.

- **Eat the rainbow.** Choose a variety of colorful fruits and vegetables to get the full range of healthful nutrients and compounds.

- **Be curious.** Don't be afraid to expand your fruit and veggie repertoire! Different cooking techniques and recipes can help you discover new favorites.

- **Stock up.** Frozen and canned fruits and vegetables are generally picked at their nutritional peak and lose almost no nutrients over time. Drain and rinse canned produce to cut down on added salt and sugar.

- **Cook smart.** Steaming and roasting are good methods to preserve nutrients. Keep cooking times short and use minimal water.

2 million people estimated that, worldwide, approximately 7.8 million premature annual deaths could be prevented if everyone ate 10 portions of fruits and vegetables per day. Even eating 2½ portions per day of fruits and vegetables was associated with an 8 percent reduction in heart-disease risk, a 16 percent reduction in stroke risk, an 8 percent reduction in cardiovascular-disease risk, and a 10 percent reduction in all-cause mortality. Even greater benefits came with higher intakes.

If you've heard that you should avoid fruit because it's mostly sugar, it's time to reconsider, because eating fruit is good for your health. Whole fruit does contain natural sugar, but it's also rich in valuable nutrients, including fiber, potassium, magnesium, folate, and vitamins A, C, and K.

Juice, on the other hand, should be approached more cautiously. It takes a while to eat and digest a whole apple because it comes packaged with fiber, which slows the release of sugar into your bloodstream. However, it only takes a minute to drink a glass of apple juice, which contains all the sugar but little-to-no fiber, which can cause a rapid spike in blood sugar. Even if you're drinking 100 percent fruit juice that contains no added sugar, consider limiting fruit juice to no more than eight ounces per day. (See Chapter 6 for more on added sugars.)

## Does Produce Have to Be Fresh?

It may come as a surprise to hear that frozen fruits and vegetables are at least as healthful as fresh and often more so. Produce that needs to travel to market is often picked early—before it's fully ripe—so it never reaches its full nutrition potential. Plus, the concentration of some nutrients lessen during shipping and storage—both in the store and in the depths of your refrigerator. Fruits and vegetables destined for freezing are fully ripened on the plant, and they're frozen and packaged within hours of harvest, preserving their peak flavor and nutritional value. Even better, they don't lose many nutrients over time.

Canned varieties can be good options, too, but they may be lower in certain nutrients because heat-sensitive vitamins like C, $B_6$, and thiamin are destroyed during the high-temperature canning process, and some of the water-soluble vitamins leach into the canning liquid. When selecting frozen or canned produce, look for fruits with no added sugar and beware of vegetables with fat- or sodium-laden sauces. The easiest way is to check the ingredients

### What Counts as a Cup of Fruit

According to MyPlate, in general, 1 cup of fruit or 100% fruit juice or ½ cup of dried fruit counts as 1 cup of fruit. See specific examples below, and learn more at ChooseMyPlate.gov.

| FRUIT | AMOUNT EQUIVALENT TO 1 CUP |
|---|---|
| Apple | • ½ large (3¼-in. diameter)<br>• 1 small (2½-in. diameter)<br>• 1 cup sliced or chopped |
| Applesauce | • 1 cup |
| Banana | • 1 cup sliced<br>• 1 large (8 to 9 in. long) |
| Grapes | • 1 cup whole or cut up<br>• 32 seedless grapes |
| Melon | • 1 cup diced or melon balls |
| Orange | • 1 large (3-in. diameter)<br>• 1 cup sections |
| Peach | • 1 large (2¾-in. diameter)<br>• 1 cup sliced, diced, or canned, drained<br>• 2 halves, canned, drained |
| Pear | • 1 medium<br>• 1 cup sliced, diced, or canned, drained |
| Plum | • 1 cup sliced<br>• 3 medium or 2 large plums |
| Dried fruit | • ½ cup |
| 100% fruit | • 1 cup |

### What Counts as a Cup of Vegetables

According to MyPlate, in general, 1 cup of raw or cooked vegetables or vegetable juice or 2 cups of raw leafy greens counts as 1 cup of vegetables. See specific examples below and learn more at ChooseMyPlate.gov.

| VEGETABLE | AMOUNT EQUIVALENT TO 1 CUP | | |
|---|---|---|---|
| Greens (such as lettuce, collard greens, kale, spinach) | • 1 cup cooked | • 2 cups raw | |
| Carrots | • 1 cup baby carrots | • 2 medium carrots | • 1 cup strips, slices, or chopped pieces |
| Bell peppers | • 1 cup chopped | • 1 large pepper | |
| Tomatoes | • 1 large tomato | • 1 cup chopped or canned | |
| Onions | • 1 cup chopped | | |
| Cucumbers | • 1 cup sliced or chopped | | |
| Potatoes | • 1 cup diced or mashed | • 1 medium boiled or baked potato (2½ to 3 in. diameter) | |
| Broccoli | • 1 cup chopped or florets | • 3 spears (5 in. long) | |
| Green beans | • 1 cup cooked | | |
| Zucchini or yellow squash | • 1 cup sliced or diced | | |

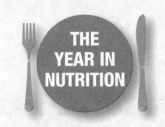

## Eat Your Leafy Greens to Keep Your Brain Sharp

Leafy green vegetables are consistently linked to better health—including protection against age-related cognitive decline. To investigate the relationship between several nutrients found in green leafy vegetables and cognitive decline, researchers followed 960 participants of the Memory and Aging project (MAP) for an average of 4.7 years. During that time, the participants, who ranged in age from 58 to 99 years, provided data on their dietary intake and underwent at least two cognitive assessment tests.

After adjusting for diet and lifestyle factors that can also affect cognitive health—for better or for worse—participants who ate the most green leafy vegetables had the lowest rate of cognitive decline. How much was "the most"? A mere 1 to 2 servings per day, on average, of spinach, lettuce salad, kale, collard greens, or other greens. According to the authors, the difference in cognitive health in this group of leafy green eaters was the equivalent of being 11 years younger. What will be in your salad tonight?

*Neurology,* January 2018

list: The healthiest options contain only one food, such as "broccoli" or "peaches."

Buying a combination of fresh, frozen, canned, and dried produce maximizes nutrition, minimizes waste, and assures that there is always a variety of fruits and vegetables on hand. When you purchase fresh fruits and vegetables, storing them appropriately can help them stay fresh and tasty longer, but if you shop just once a week, keeping canned and frozen produce on hand can save you money because you won't be throwing out limp or rotting produce you didn't get around to eating.

## Necessary to Choose Organic or Not?

Many people are surprised to learn that organic produce is not necessarily more nutritious than conventionally grown produce. The most nutritious fruits and vegetables, organic or not, are the ones that have reached peak ripeness on the plant and are eaten as close to harvest as possible. The difference with organic foods

## Storing Fresh Fruits and Vegetables for Best Flavor

### STORE IN THE REFRIGERATOR

| Fruit | | Vegetables | |
|---|---|---|---|
| • Apples (more than 7 days) | • Artichokes | • Cauliflower | • Lettuce |
| • Apricots | • Asparagus | • Celery | • Mushrooms |
| • Asian Pears | • Green Beans | • Cut Vegetables | • Peas |
| • Berries | • Beets | • Green Onions | • Radishes |
| • Cherries | • Belgian Endive | • Herbs (not basil) | • Spinach |
| • Cut Fruit | • Broccoli | • Leafy Vegetables | • Sprouts |
| • Figs | • Brussels Sprouts | | • Summer Squash |
| • Grapes | • Cabbage | • Leeks | • Sweet Corn |
| | • Carrots | | |

1. Place fruits and vegetables in separate, perforated plastic bags.
2. Use within 1 to 3 days for maximum flavor and freshness.
3. Store fruits and vegetables in different refrigerator drawers. Some fruits produce a gas called ethylene glycol that hastens ripening, causing spoilage in some vegetables.

### ALLOW TO RIPEN ON THE COUNTER, THEN REFRIGERATE

| | | | |
|---|---|---|---|
| • Avocados | • Nectarines | • Pears | • Plumcots |
| • Kiwi | • Peaches | • Plums | |

1. To prevent moisture loss, store fruits and vegetables separately in a paper bag, perforated plastic bag, or ripening bowl on the counter away from sunlight. Speed up ripening of fruit in a bowl or paper bag by placing an apple with the fruit to be ripened.
2. After ripening, store in refrigerator and use within 1 to 3 days.

### STORE ONLY AT ROOM TEMPERATURE

| Fruit | | Vegetables | |
|---|---|---|---|
| • Apples (fewer than 7 days) | • Papayas | • Basil (in water) | • Peppers* |
| • Bananas | • Persimmons | • Cucumber* | • Potatoes** |
| • Citrus Fruits | • Pineapple | • Eggplant* | • Pumpkins |
| • Mangoes | • Plantain | • Garlic** | • Sweet Potatoes** |
| • Melons | • Pomegranates | • Ginger | • Tomatoes |
| | | • Jicama | • Winter Squashes |
| | | • Onions** | |

1. Many fruits and vegetables should only be stored at room temperature. Refrigeration can cause cold damage or prevent them from ripening to good flavor and texture.
2. Keep away from direct sunlight.

*Cucumbers, eggplant, and peppers can be refrigerated for 1 to 3 days if they are used soon after removing from the refrigerator.
**Store garlic, onions, potatoes, and sweet potatoes in a well-ventilated area in the pantry.

Source: Produce for Better Health Foundation (FruitsAndVeggiesMoreMatters.org)

lies in the types of pesticides used and the fact that they have not undergone genetic modification. Organic agriculture also may have benefits for the environment.

If you're concerned about pesticides in your produce, use the Pesticide Residue Calculator at SafeFruitsandVeggies.com. It's important to remember that the health benefits of eating fruits and vegetables likely outweigh any dangers from chemical residues. If organic produce is unavailable or too costly, scrubbing conventional produce before eating it is a good option to remove any residual pesticides. The Food and Drug Administration (FDA) points out that washing all fresh produce, whether conventional or organically grown, before eating it is a healthful habit. To reduce, or even eliminate, any pesticide residues present on fresh fruits and vegetables, as well as dirt or bacteria, the agency recommends following these simple tips:

- **Wash produce** with large amounts of cold or warm tap water, scrubbing with a brush if appropriate, but do not use soap.
- **Throw away the outer leaves** of leafy vegetables, such as lettuce and cabbage.
- **Don't forget to clean your hands,** scrub brushes, and colanders before using them to wash your fresh produce.

## Health-Promoting Compounds

Study after study shows that higher fruit and vegetable intake is linked to lower chronic disease risk. What makes these foods so powerful? Certainly, the healthful vitamins and minerals play an important role, coupled with the fact that these foods are full of fiber, but plant foods also deliver a variety of health-promoting substances called phytochemicals (also called phytonutrients). The term "phytochemicals" covers thousands of nutrients that deliver a wide range of health benefits to our bodies. The color of a fruit or vegetable often hints at its nutrients, especially the phytochemicals it contains. For example,

carotenoids (such as beta-carotene, lutein, and lycopene) give carrots, tomatoes, and watermelon their yellow, orange, and red hues, while anthocyanins provide the deep red, purple, and blue hues in berries, purple cabbage, and black rice.

Some phytochemicals function as antioxidants. Antioxidants neutralize free radicals, compounds that can damage cells and tissues and induce inflammation. Thus, these phytochemicals can minimize cell damage from free radicals, helping to keep cells healthy and reduce systemic inflammation and the risk of diseases such as cancer and cardiovascular disease. Other nutrients found in fruits and vegetables such as vitamins C and E, which are not phytochemicals, also have antioxidant properties. Phytochemicals can also be beneficial to the immune system and help support gut health.

Eating whole fruits and vegetables, rather than taking isolated phytochemical supplements, can potentially lead to greater health benefits because phytochemicals act synergistically with each other and with vitamins, minerals, and other nutrients in foods.

Different phytochemicals and nutrients provide different health benefits, so the best way to make sure you're getting plenty of these powerful compounds is to diversify your fruit and vegetable "portfolio." Creating a rainbow of colors on your plate will maximize the variety of phytochemicals in your diet.

## The Weight Connection

Another way fruits and vegetables may reduce risk of disease and premature death is through their impact on body weight. Research suggests that including plenty of fruits and non-starchy vegetables in your eating plan may help you to reach and maintain a healthy weight. Another benefit to eating more fruits and vegetables is that there is less room on your plate for less healthful foods. Additionally, the dietary

**SMART SHIFT**

### Eat Fruits and Vegetables Throughout the Day

Upping your fruit and vegetable intake is a great way to increase your intake of health-promoting vitamins, minerals, fiber, and phytochemicals. Fitting these nutrition powerhouses into every meal and snack is a great goal for anyone looking to support their long-term health. Try these simple suggestions to shift your diet toward fruits and vegetables:

**BREAKFAST**
- Top cereal with fruit
- Eat berries with yogurt or kefir
- Stuff an omelet with sautéed vegetables
- Choose a side of fruit instead of potatoes
- Grab fruit with yogurt and/or a (low sugar) snack bar to go

**LUNCH**
- Load sandwiches with vegetables
- Choose a side of fruit or veggies instead of fries or chips
- Throw leftovers over greens for a satisfying salad
- Toss last night's veggies with grains and a drizzle of dressing
- Finish with fruit

**DINNER**
- Put salad on your plate
- Build your meal around the veggies on hand
- Load soups, stews, casseroles, chili, and pasta dishes with extra veggies
- Buy pre-cut veggies (or prep your own) to make using them convenient

**SNACKS/TREATS**
- Grab a sweet, juicy fruit
- Dip veggies in hummus, nut butter, or salsa
- Grill peach halves or pineapple slices
- Bake apples
- Dip fruit slices in nut butter
- Snack on a handful of dried fruit with nuts

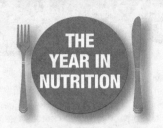

## More Flavonoids, More Favorable Health?

Fruits and vegetables. Green tea. Cocoa. Red wine. Each comes "packaged" with a lot of attributed health benefits and claims about disease prevention. In a recent systematic review and meta-analysis of 22 studies, researchers took a closer look at a few specific components that these foods and beverages have in common to elicit what role they might play in health and longevity.

The authors found that a higher intake of flavonoids was associated with lower risk of death from cardiovascular disease and all other causes. While most types of flavonoids appeared to protect against cardiovascular-related death, three types—flavones, flavanones, and anthocyanidins— were linked to lower risk of death from all causes.

The authors hypothesized that these benefits likely come from flavonoids' antioxidant and anti-inflammatory benefits, which may reduce the risk of many chronic diseases, including cardiovascular disease and cancer. All the more reason to enjoy a variety of vegetables and fruits— especially anthocyanidin-rich berries—and relax with a cup of flavanol-rich green tea!

*American Journal of Epidemiology,* June 2017

fiber and water in fruits and vegetables take up more space in your stomach, giving you a greater feeling of fullness and possibly preventing overeating. The dietary fiber and other complex carbohydrates found in fruits and vegetables also provide food for the good bacteria that live in your colon. When your gut bacteria feast on fiber, they produce short-chain fatty acids. These fatty acids may help promote satiety (the feeling that you've eaten enough), keep hunger in check, and reduce inflammation. Scientific research on the role of gut bacteria on health continues to evolve, but we already know that eating a variety of fruits and vegetables—along with other plant foods—is good for gut health.

## Upping Your Intake

Every dietary pattern discussed in Chapter 2 recommends eating fruits and vegetables throughout the day, with at least half a plate's worth at every meal. This is not as difficult as it may sound: Simply add a serving of your favorite vegetable, a side salad, or toss extra veggies in your pasta dishes and casseroles. Soups and stews are great places to sneak in some extra vegetables, and nothing beats a big, no-cooking-required salad with greens, veggies, protein (canned beans or tuna if you don't have any leftovers), and nuts or seeds on a hot day. Choosing fruit for your weekday dessert is a satisfying and nutritious way to end a meal.

How you store and cook vegetables affects their nutritional value, taste, and texture. Exposure to heat reduces levels of some nutrients but makes other nutrients more available, so vegetables are a healthful choice either raw or cooked. Many people think they don't like vegetables or limit themselves to a few regular choices, but the taste and texture of vegetables can change dramatically depending on how they're cooked. For example, some people don't like boiled Brussels sprouts but love how roasting makes them sweet and tender. Try different recipes and cooking techniques before giving up on a vegetable entirely.

Fruits and vegetables are packed with proven health-promoting vitamins, minerals, fiber, and phytochemicals, and they're low in calories. To reap the most benefits from fruits and vegetables, include them— raw, cooked, frozen, canned, or dried—at every meal and snack throughout the day.

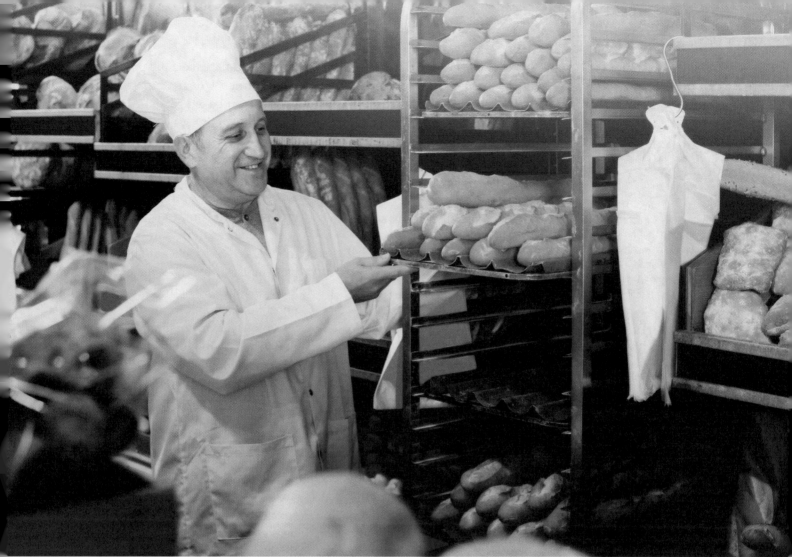

## 4  Fill Up with Fiber

Grains and legumes sometimes get a bad rap. For some, it's because of the belief that carbohydrates cause weight gain. For others, it's because of the idea that humans didn't evolve to eat agriculture-based foods like grains and legumes. Yes, whole grains and legumes (beans, lentils, peas, and soybeans) contain carbohydrates (which we really do need), but they also provide quality plant-based protein. Even better, they are packed with dietary fiber and nutrients, including B vitamins to help keep your metabolism running well and antioxidants to help protect your cells from damage. Plus, whole grains and legumes are integral parts of many traditional diets from around the world, including those that are associated with better health and a longer life.

### Grains

Grains (also known as cereals) are the fruits (seeds) of grasses. The latest *Dietary Guidelines for Americans* say that people who eat 2,000 calories per day can eat six ounce-equivalent servings of grains daily, but at least half of these servings should be whole grains. In general, one ounce-equivalent is a slice of bread, 1 cup of ready-to-eat cereal, or ½ cup of cooked pasta, rice, oatmeal, or other grains.

The term "whole grain" refers to the entire grain seed as it grows in nature. Whole wheat, whole corn, oats, brown rice, quinoa, sorghum, and rye berries are some examples of whole grains. All whole grain foods or ingredients consist of three parts:

▶ **The bran,** the outer layer that protects the seed, is an excellent source of fiber. It

"Whole grain" bread means the entire grain seed is included in the bread, something bakeries are including in their offerings.

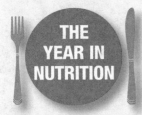

**THE YEAR IN NUTRITION**

### Dietary Fiber Is Good for Heart Health

When people think about fiber and health, they typically think about digestive health. Yes, consuming adequate dietary fiber can help "keep you regular," but a recent study concluded that fiber is important for many more health reasons—including heart health.

The "umbrella study" of 18 previously published meta-analyses—which themselves covered 298 separate observational studies—found evidence that a higher intake of dietary fiber is associated with a lower risk of cardiovascular disease, type 2 diabetes, and some forms of cancer. The strongest evidence was for a reduced risk of cardiovascular disease, especially coronary artery disease (heart disease) and death from cardiovascular disease. The authors said this may be because dietary fiber can promote healthier cholesterol levels.

While not as strong, there was "suggestive evidence" that dietary fiber may lower the risk of type 2 diabetes and pancreatic cancer. This may be because dietary fiber may help reduce chronic inflammation—a factor in cancer, diabetes, cardiovascular disease, and other health conditions—and promote stable blood sugar levels. Fiber-rich fruits, vegetables, whole-grains, and legumes are also rich in a wide array of nutrients that are beneficial to health. Increasing your intake of these foods will boost your daily fiber intake—so fill up!

*American Journal of Clinical Nutrition,* March 2018

**DIETLIFE TIPS**

▶ **Make half your grains whole grain.** Replacing at least half of the refined-grain foods or products you eat with whole grains will improve your overall diet quality.

▶ **Enjoy legumes.** Beans, lentils, and peas are packed with fiber, protein, and other health-promoting nutrients.

▶ **Toss in nuts and seeds** to add fiber plus healthy fats (see chapter 7) to salads, trail mixes, and breakfast cereals.

▶ **Substitute, don't add.** Eat a variety of healthy foods, making sure to swap out those less healthy choices.

is also rich in B vitamins, which play an important role in metabolism and energy production and support the normal functioning of the nervous system.

▶ **The germ** is the inner portion of the grain, or the seed's embryo, that can grow into a new plant. The germ contains antioxidants (including vitamin E) and other phytochemicals, B vitamins, important minerals such as iron and magnesium, some protein, and healthy fats.

▶ **The endosperm** is the largest part of the grain. It's composed primarily of protein and starchy carbohydrates, which provide energy to the growing plant.

Whole grains are generally high in fiber, iron, potassium, phosphorus, magnesium, zinc, calcium, B vitamins, and vitamin E, and they contain a variety of phytochemicals. The term "refined grains" refers to whole grains that have been processed to remove the nutrient-rich bran and germ layer, leaving only the starchy endosperm. This includes, for example, turning whole-wheat flour into refined white flour or converting brown rice into white rice. While Americans don't eat enough whole grains, they eat too many refined grains, especially products made from refined wheat flour (white bread, pasta, sweet baked goods). Almost half of the refined grains we eat are from mixed dishes, such as burgers, sandwiches, pizza, burritos, macaroni and cheese, and pasta dishes.

The process of refining whole wheat into what is commonly called "white flour" removes most of the vitamins and minerals. Refined wheat flour provides 19 percent less protein, 75 percent less fiber, and less than half of the iron, magnesium, phosphorus, potassium, zinc, niacin, and vitamin $B_6$ than a cup of whole-wheat flour. The FDA requires that several B vitamins and iron be added back into refined flour to prevent nutrient deficiencies in the population, resulting in what is known as "enriched flour." However, many of the other beneficial nutrients and phytochemicals are still missing. Diets rich in whole grains are associated with a variety of health benefits.

Another large study found a number of health benefits linked to a diet in which the majority of grains are whole: reduction in risks of death from any cause (17 percent), cancer (15 percent), respiratory disease (22 percent), diabetes (51 percent), and infectious disease (26 percent), along with substantially lower risks of cardiovascular disease and stroke. Inflammation plays a role in many of these conditions, and whole grains may have anti-inflammatory effects. Results of a clinical trial conducted by Tufts University researchers and published in 2017 found that adults who consumed a diet rich in whole grains, rather than refined grains, had an increase in bacteria that produce short-chain fatty acids (SCFAs). These SCFAs play important roles in reducing inflammation and decreasing bacteria that increase inflammation. Increasing our intake of whole-grains may influence the composition of our gut microbes and thus improve our health by reducing inflammation.

Whole grains may even help you maintain a healthy weight. A number of observational studies have found that people who eat two to three servings of whole grains per day have smaller waist circumferences (less abdominal fat) compared with those who eat few or no whole grains. The dietary fiber in whole grains may play a role by reducing the rate of digestion and prolonging a feeling of fullness. But it's important to keep in mind that evidence suggests the benefits to your waistline from eating more whole grains are reduced if you continue to eat too many refined grains, such as white bread, white rice, and pastries, so be sure to choose whole grains in place of refined grains, rather than just adding them.

## Shift to Whole Grains

Clearly, shifting an eating pattern to replace refined grains with whole grains will improve the nutritional quality of your diet and improve your overall health. You can increase your whole-grain intake by eating more whole-grain products, such as whole-wheat breads and pastas, and more intact (not milled into flour) whole grains. Brown rice and oats (and even popcorn) are common intact whole grains, and there are many delicious alternatives that are less familiar but gaining in popularity. If eating three servings of whole grains seems daunting to you, start by switching out one refined-grain food for a whole-grain version.

It's relatively easy to replace refined grains with whole-grain options. For example, start the day with steel-cut oatmeal instead of refined cold cereals at breakfast, use whole-grain bread at lunch, have popcorn instead of chips for a snack, and serve whole grains as a side dish at dinner. Eating brown rice in place of white rice is one option, but consider trying other grains, too. Try barley in place of rice as a side dish. Quinoa is quick and easy to cook and very versatile, good in hot side dishes, cold salads, or even stirred into soups or chilis. It's one of the rare plant foods that contain all the essential amino acids. Quinoa also is high in potassium, which can help lower blood pressure and has an unusually high ratio of protein to carbohydrates for a grain. Just be sure to rinse it before cooking to wash away the bitter saponins that protect the seeds from pests in the wild.

### What Counts as a Serving of Grains

It is recommended that adults consume 5 to 7 servings (called ounce-equivalents) of grains per day, depending on their calorie needs. Below are a few examples of what counts as a serving of grains.

| GRAIN | 1 SERVING (OUNCE-EQUIVALENT) OF GRAINS |
|---|---|
| Bagels | • 1 mini bagel |
| Breads | • 1 regular slice |
| Bulgur | • ½ cup cooked |
| Crackers | • 5 whole-wheat crackers<br>• 2 rye crispbreads<br>• 7 square or round crackers |
| English muffins | • ½ muffin |
| Oatmeal | • ½ cup cooked<br>• 1 packet instant<br>• ⅓ cup dry |
| Popcorn | • 3 cups, popped |
| Pasta or rice | • ½ cup cooked; 1 ounce uncooked |
| Ready-to-eat breakfast cereals | • 1 cup, flakes or rounds<br>• 1¼ cups puffed |
| Tortilla | • 1 corn or flour tortilla (6 in. diameter) |

Aim to make at least half of your grain servings whole-grain foods. Look for the Whole Grains Stamp on packaged foods to find out how many grams of whole grains are in the serving size listed on the label. Your goal is at least 48 grams of whole grains a day.

### Evaluating the Whole-Grain Content of Packaged Foods

- In all food ingredient lists, the first item on the list makes up the highest percentage of the product. Look for products with a whole grain listed as the first or second ingredient. Whole-grain ingredients also include wheat berries, brown rice, oats, oatmeal, and sprouted grains (a refined grain can't be sprouted).

- Terms like "enriched wheat" and "degerminated corn" on labels indicate refined grains. That means these are NOT whole-grain products. "Wheat," "semolina wheat," and "durum wheat" also are likely to be refined grains unless they have the word "whole" in front of them. "Multigrain" products don't necessarily contain whole grains (they might be made from multiple refined grains), so check the ingredient list.

- Look for fiber. Since whole grains are a source of dietary fiber, look for at least 1 gram (g) of fiber for each 10 g of total carbohydrate. But, keep in mind that whole-grain products that contain less fiber are still more nutritious than their refined-grain counterparts.

- If the product contains at least 16 grams of whole grains and no refined grains, it may bear a "100% Whole Grain" stamp from the Whole Grains Council. Food manufacturers have to pay a fee to participate in this program, so not all whole-grain products bear the stamp. The daily goal for whole grains is at least 48 grams, which is equivalent to three servings of whole grains. Keep in mind that this stamp only appears on processed foods (those in boxes or bags), which may be high in added fats, sugars, and calories. Learn more about the Whole Grain Stamp at wholegrainscouncil.org.

| Your Guide to Whole Grains | | Cooking | | | |
|---|---|---|---|---|---|
| From amaranth to wild rice, here's a primer on the many whole-grain options that are available. | | Start with 1 cup of these intact whole grains, rinsed: | | | |
| GRAINS | | GLUTEN FREE | ADD WATER: | BRING TO A BOIL, THEN SIMMER FOR:** | COOKED YIELD |
| Amaranth | Tiny beige seeds that cook up into a delicate, slightly gelatinous porridge. | yes* | 3 c | 20 to 25 min. | 2 c |
| Brown rice | Short, medium, and long-grain varieties are available. | yes* | 2½ c | 25 to 45 min. | 3-4 c |
| Buckwheat | The whole buckwheat kernels (which are actually seeds) are shaped a bit like a pyramid; when roasted, they have a hearty, nutty flavor. | yes* | 2 c | 20 min. | 4 c |
| Cornmeal (polenta) | Ground, dried corn kernels. Be sure to choose stone-ground whole-grain cornmeal, which retains some of the hull and germ of the corn. Regular cornmeal has been degermed and is not a whole grain. | yes* | 4 c | 25 to 30 min. | 2½ c |
| Barley (hulled) | Barley kernels are intact, but the outer (inedible) husk has been removed. | no | 3 c | 45 to 60 min. | 3½ c |
| Millet (hulled) | Small yellow kernels that cook up into a dish that has a texture somewhere between a pilaf and porridge. | yes* | 2 c | 25 to 35 min. | 2½ c |
| Oat groats | The entire kernel of the grain, minus the inedible outer husk. | yes* | 3 c | 50 to 60 min. | 3 c |
| Quinoa | Tiny seeds with a delicate flavor. Typically ivory in color, but red and black varieties also are available. | yes* | 2 c | 12 to 15 min | 4 c |
| Rolled oats | Oat groats that have been steamed and flattened to produce rolled oats. Look for "old-fashioned" or regular oats, not quick or instant. | yes* | 2 c | 5 minutes | 2 c |
| Rye berries | Whole kernels of rye with the inedible hull removed. | no | 4 c | 45 to 60 min. | 3 c |
| Sorghum | Unlike some grains, sorghum doesn't have an inedible outer hull, so it's often eaten with all of its nutritious, outer layers. | yes* | 3 c | 45 to 60 min. | 2½ c |
| Steel-cut oats | Oat groats that have been cut into several pieces with steel blades (hence the term "steel-cut"). | yes* | 4 c | 20 to 30 min. | 4 c |
| Teff | Minuscule beige or brown seeds. Originally from Ethiopia. Available in whole grain or flour form. | yes* | 3 c | 20 min. | 2½ c |
| Wild rice | Although not a true grain or rice but an aquatic grass, it offers similar nutritional benefits to whole grains. | yes* | 3 c | 45 to 55 min. | 3½ c |
| WHEAT: Numerous varieties of wheat in various forms beyond flour are available. All wheat products contain gluten. | | | | | |
| Bulgur | Whole-wheat kernels that have been steamed, dried, and cracked. | no | 2 c | 10 to 15 min. | 3 c |
| Cracked wheat | Wheat berries that have been broken into small pieces. Do not confuse with bulgur. | no | 3 c | 15 to 20 min. | 3 c |
| Farro (Emmer) | An ancient wheat variety, farro is believed to have sustained the Roman legions. | no | 3 c | 30 to 45 min. | 2 c |
| Kamut | A hardy ancient type of wheat originally from the Fertile Crescent. | no | 3 c | 45 to 60 min. | 3 c |
| Spelt | An ancient subspecies of wheat that packs its nutrition in the inner kernel rather than in exterior bran and germ layers as in traditional wheat. | no | 3 c | 65 to 80 min. | 2¼ c |
| Wheat berries | Whole kernels of wheat that have had outer husks removed. Chewy texture and nutty flavor. | no | 3 c | 60 min | 3 c |

Note: c = cups, min. = minutes.

*Check packages for a statement certifying that the grain is free of gluten if you are gluten intolerant. Oats and some other gluten-free grains may be contaminated with gluten unless specifically marked gluten-free.

**You can reduce cooking time by soaking intact whole grains overnight. Cooking times can vary, so cook until tender. If needed, add more water during cooking.

Adults should aim to eat 5 to 7 servings (or ounce equivalents) of grains per day, at least half of them whole. Packaged foods that contain whole grains are often marked with the Whole Grain Stamp created by the Whole Grains Council. This stamp tells you how many grams of whole grain are in the product. If you're eating processed foods made with flour, keep in mind that whole-grain options can still be high in added sugars and/or saturated fat. For example, whole-grain muffins, although better than their refined-grain counterparts, may contain a lot of sugar and/or saturated fat and should be eaten in moderation. While popcorn is a whole-grain food, skip the sugar-coated, cheesy, and buttery varieties. To sleuth out how many whole grains are in a processed food, it's important to look at the ingredient list and the Nutrition Facts Panel and not just rely on phrases like "made with whole grains" on the front of the bag or box.

## Legumes

Legumes are the seeds of plants in the pea family; they include pulses (see below), green peas, soybeans, and peanuts. Research suggests that legumes may help lower both total and unhealthy (LDL) cholesterol, reduce blood pressure, and help control blood sugar. Some research has linked eating beans to a reduced risk of colon cancer, possibly because the fiber in beans helps to support healthy bacteria in the large intestine. Eating beans, which are legumes, also has been linked with longevity. Legumes provide protein, iron, zinc, fiber, potassium, and folate, among other nutrients. They also satisfy hunger just as well as meat-based meals, according to research from

**Whole Grain Stamp**

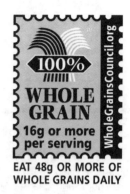

### Nutrients in Whole, Refined, and Enriched Wheat

Whole-wheat kernels are stripped of their bran and germ before being ground into refined wheat flour. This removes many vitamins and minerals, fiber, and some protein. Refined wheat flour is required by law to be enriched by replacing some of the lost vitamins and minerals. This graphic, courtesy of the Whole Grains Council, demonstrates the balanced nutrition of whole grains, as opposed to refined or enriched.

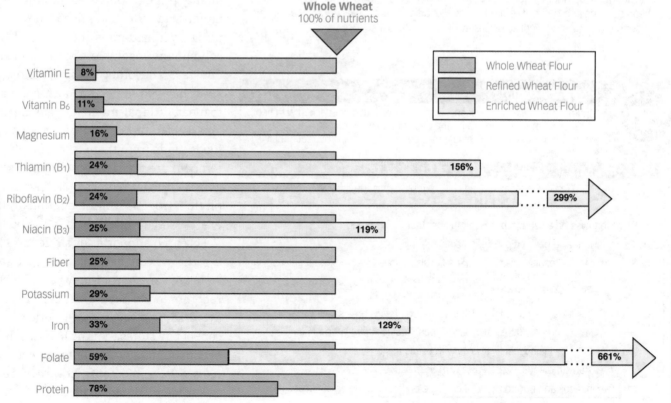

Image Courtesy of Oldways Whole Grain Council

the University of Copenhagen in Denmark. Most adults should have at least 1½ cups of legumes per week. Unfortunately, only 8 percent of adults living in the United States eat legumes on any given day, even though they are great in soups, stews, salads, and salsas, or as an entrée on their own.

## Have You Tried Farro?

Farro is an ancient form of wheat that's hearty and robust, with a natural sweetness and pleasant chewiness that lends itself well to a variety of dishes, including pilafs, soups, and salads. Enjoyed by Italians for centuries, it provided sustenance for the ancient Roman legions. Wild emmer (farro) dates back 17,000 years to the late Paleolithic era and was first domesticated about 10,000 years ago in the Fertile Crescent.

Farro soup with beans, chickpeas, greens, and maybe seafood is a well-known Tuscan dish. The risotto-like dish "farrotto" benefits from a starch found in emmer farro that is similar to the starch in Arborio rice. In Italy, farro refers to three types of ancient wheat: einkorn *(farro piccolo)*, emmer *(farro medio),* and spelt *(farro grande)*. Technically speaking, however, emmer is the true farro.

Although most farro sold in the United States is emmer, spelt, and einkorn are sometimes labeled as farro. That can make estimating cooking time a challenge, as can the fact that emmer farro may be sold whole, semi-pearled (some of the bran has been removed) or pearled (all of the bran has been removed). Pearled and semi-pearled farro cook in about 20 to 30 minutes, while true whole grain farro can take 45 to 60 minutes. For each cup of farro, add 2 cups of water. You also can cook farro using the pasta method, using at least 4 cups of water per cup of farro.

Farro and other ancient wheats are higher in soluble fiber and protein than standard wheat. Compared with modern wheat, farro is higher in fiber, protein, and certain antioxidants and minerals. Farro tends to contain less gluten than common bread wheat, so it may be better tolerated by individuals with non-celiac gluten sensitivity, although individuals with celiac disease will need to avoid it.

### SMART SHIFT

## Swap in Legumes

Legumes (beans, peas, soybeans, lentils, and peanuts) are packed with fiber, protein, and other health-promoting nutrients. To meet recommendations, aim to eat at least 1½ cups of legumes per week. To help you reach that goal, try these tips:

| INSTEAD OF... | TRY... |
| --- | --- |
| Chili with meat | Bean chili, or replace half the meat with beans |
| Pasta salad | Lentil salad |
| Mayonnaise on a sandwich | Hummus or other bean spread |
| Creamy or mayonnaise-based dips | Bean dips |
| Regular salsa | Black-bean salsa or beans stirred into regular salsa |
| Potato chips or pretzels | Steamed edamame (green soybeans in the pod) or roasted chickpeas |
| Meat on a salad | Chickpeas or other beans on a salad |
| Cream soups | Lentil, split pea, or black-bean soup |
| Plain grains | Grains with beans |
| Pasta with meat sauce | Pasta with bean sauce |
| Meat in tacos and burritos | Replace some or all of the meat with beans |

A large subgroup of the legume family is pulses, which include lentils, chickpeas (garbanzo beans), black-eyed peas, split peas, kidney beans, pinto beans, black beans, and many other bean varieties.

Typically, you can buy pulses dried or canned. If you buy canned, choose no-salt-added or low-sodium varieties, or drain and rinse them, which will wash away about 40 percent of the sodium. One benefit of cooking dried beans is that they have little sodium unless you add salt. Some people may avoid legumes because they feel these fiber-rich foods cause gut discomfort and gas. To reduce some of the gas-producing compounds in beans, soak them longer than required, discard the water, and cook them in fresh water. Your body also tends to adjust, so the more often you eat legumes, the less uncomfortable you are likely to be.

## The Scoop on Soy Foods

One bean that stands out is the soybean. Whether eaten right out of the pod (edamame), roasted (soy nuts), or made into tofu or tempeh, soybeans are a high-quality protein source, containing all the amino acids our bodies need. They're also packed with vitamins and minerals, have soluble and insoluble fiber, and provide omega-3 and omega-6 fatty acids. Soy foods have no cholesterol and, compared to meat, little saturated fat, making them an excellent protein source. Soybeans and foods made from them (such as tofu and tempeh) are the richest source of isoflavones in the human diet. (Isoflavones are phytoestrogens—plant chemicals that exert estrogen-like effects in the body.)

Research supports soy's role in reducing the risk of osteoporosis and some forms of cancer. For many years, doctors recommended breast-cancer survivors avoid soy; however, the American Cancer Society states that the health benefits of consuming soy appear to outweigh any risks. Soy supplements, however, are not recommended. Since 1999, the FDA has allowed soy-food products to carry the authorized health claim that soy protein reduces heart-disease risk, but that claim is being reevaluated in light of newer evidence suggesting that the link between soy protein and heart health is weaker than previously thought.

Include protein-rich edamame (immature green soybeans that are tender and sweet), mature soybeans (black, white, or crispy toasted), and soy products such as tofu and tempeh in your healthy dietary pattern.

## Fabulous Fiber

Plant foods offer a range of different types of fiber. It is recommended that women ages 19 to 50 aim for a daily fiber intake (i.e. adequate intake) of at least 25 grams, and 21 grams for women over 50. The adequate intake for men ages 19 to 50 years old is 38 grams, and 30 grams for men over 50. Unfortunately, the fiber intake of the average American adult is only about 15 grams per day, so most people are missing out on the tremendous health benefits that fiber can provide.

In addition to helping prevent constipation, diets rich in dietary fiber have been associated with lower blood lipid levels and blood pressure, reduced inflammation, weight loss, and increased immune function and glucose control. Fiber also feeds the beneficial bacteria that inhabit our digestive systems. Different types of fiber exert different health-promoting effects on the body, so eating a variety of fiber-rich foods will help you gain the most benefits. Because fiber is a hot nutritional topic, especially as researchers learn more about the gut microbiota, many food manufacturers are putting added fibers in foods. While some research shows that added fibers have benefit, it varies based on the fiber. And some foods with added

### Benefits of Fiber

Numerous randomized controlled clinical trials in people with type 2 diabetes have found that fiber helps improve blood sugar control, as well as cholesterol and triglyceride levels.

Viscous fibers, such as those found in oats and legumes, can lower LDL cholesterol levels and help with blood sugar control.

Fiber may help prevent weight gain or promote weight loss. Since fiber cannot be broken down and absorbed by the body, high-fiber foods have less calories. There is also some evidence that eating foods with fiber will help you feel full for longer periods of time.

Some dietary fibers are classified as *prebiotic*—they provide food for the beneficial bacteria that live in your gut. Since different gut microbes like to munch on different kinds of fiber, studies suggest the more fiber you consume from a wide range of plant foods, the more diverse your gut microbiota will be, and this is important to health.

When the helpful bacteria ferment fiber in your gut, they produce short-chain fatty acids (SCFAs). SCFAs are known to support the immune system and help preserve gut health, and they may have anti-inflammatory roles in our bodies.

### Have You Tried Lentils?

Lentils are a type of "pulse," the edible seeds of legumes, along with beans, peas, and chickpeas. Lentils come in different sizes, shapes, and colors. You're most likely to find large green lentils and split red lentils in the grocery store. Split lentils cook faster than whole lentils and are great in curries, as a soup thickener, and even in smoothies, while whole lentils work better in salads and other dishes where you need them to retain their shape and texture. Other types of whole lentils that are becoming more popular are black Beluga lentils (sometimes called Caviar lentils) and French green lentils (sometimes called Puy lentils). While whole lentils, compared to split lentils, take longer to cook, they both cook more quickly than dried beans. Something to think about if you're in a hurry!

To speed up dinner prep time, you can cook a big batch of lentils and freeze them in meal-size portions for up to three months. Refrigerated leftovers last for one week. Dried lentils keep in your cool, dry cupboard or pantry for up to a year. Once you open the original packaging, transfer them to an airtight container.

You'll have an opportunity to get to know green lentils with three very different recipes in the seven-day menu plan at the end of the book: Broccoli and Lentil Salad, the Lentil-Walnut Spread, and Shrimp with White Wine, Lentils, and Tomatoes. Enjoy this tiny, but mighty, pulse!

fiber are less-than-healthy. Foods that are naturally fiber-rich come as part of a complete nutritional package. Not only do you get their intrinsic fiber, but you get a host of naturally occurring vitamins, minerals, and phytonutrients. Just some food for thought!

Many of us choose to get our protein from meat, preferably served with a variety of vegetables and grains.

- **Limit red meat.** Aim for fewer than four three-ounce servings per week. Examples of red meat are beef, pork, bison, lamb, goat, and game meat, such as elk and venison.

- **Avoid processed meats.** Often high in saturated fat, sodium, and nitrates, processed meats like sausage, bacon, ham, hot dogs, salami, bologna, and beef jerky have been linked to cancer.

- **Choose lean cuts.** Lean cuts are often signaled by the words "loin" and "round," such as "eye of round" or "tenderloin."

- **Switch animal proteins.** Enjoy fish/seafood, poultry, and low-fat or fat-free dairy products more often.

- **Eat more fish and seafood.** Fish and seafood in general are an excellent protein source. Aim for at least two servings (about 8 oz.) of fish or seafood per week.

- **Pick plant proteins.** Fit beans or lentils—this includes soy foods—into your diet at least twice weekly as a healthful protein source, and don't forget grains (especially quinoa). Nuts and seeds also provide protein.

- **Don't make meat the focal point.** Use smaller amounts of meat as an ingredient in dishes. For instance, use a bit of meat in vegetable-rich soup, stir-fry dishes, or to top a salad.

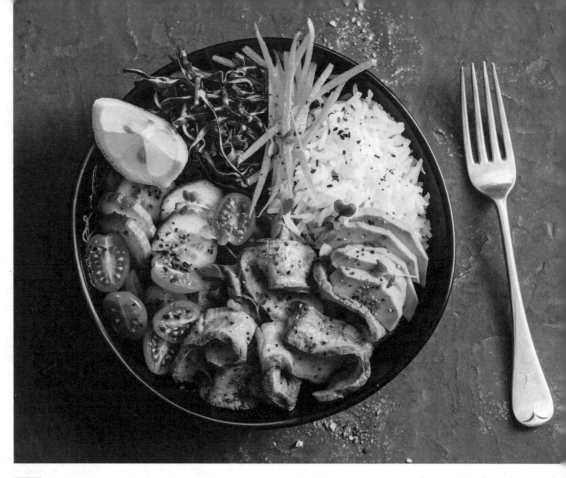

## 5 Power Up with Proteins

What do you know about protein? You probably know that your muscles are made of protein, and you might know (or have noticed) that getting enough protein with meals helps you stay satisfied longer. But protein is so much more than that. Your bones, skin, hair, fingernails, and other body tissues are made of protein, and so are your hormones, enzymes, and immune-system antibodies. A special protein called hemoglobin transports oxygen through your blood to all corners of your body.

Hemoglobin is just one of the more than 10,000 proteins in the human body. Each protein is built from a different combination of 20 amino acids, nine of which we need to get from food (the essential amino acids). Animal-based protein foods (including seafood, poultry, beef, pork, lamb, eggs, and dairy) contain all nine. Most plant-based protein sources are missing or are low in one or two essential amino acids. Only soy, quinoa, buckwheat, and amaranth are the exceptions. But the good news is that you can build an eating plan based on other plant proteins like beans, lentils, peas, whole grains, and nuts and seeds and still get all the amino acids you need. Just include a variety of foods over the course of the day—there's no need to do "old school" food combining like pairing rice and beans to "make" a complete protein.

### Protein Recommendations

In the MyPlate graphics, protein takes up one-quarter of the plate. Following this visual advice will help you achieve the 5 to 6½ ounce-equivalents of daily protein recommended by the USDA. Each ounce-equivalent of animal protein, such as meat, fish, or eggs, provides about 7 grams of protein; ounce-equivalents of plant-based proteins are more variable. For example, ½ ounce of almonds and ¼ cup of cooked black beans each have about 3 grams of protein, and ¼ cup of roasted soybeans has 10 grams of protein.

You also can calculate your minimum protein intake based on body weight. In general, the Recommended Dietary Allowance (RDA) for protein is 0.8 grams of protein per kilogram of body weight (0.37 grams per pound) for healthy adults. So, a 160-pound person would need about 60 grams of protein per day (160 multiplied by 0.37 equals 60). Again, not all this daily protein intake will need to come from animal sources. Simply eating the recommended servings of grains and vegetables provides over 20 grams of protein. In fact, if your diet were composed entirely of plant foods, you would still be able to consume adequate protein. Although people commonly eat more than enough protein at dinner, breakfast typically falls short.

Many people believe that a low-protein diet is necessary for slowing the progression of chronic kidney disease (CKD), but a 2017 study found that replacing even one serving of red or processed meat with a serving of legumes, low-fat dairy, fish/seafood, or nuts reduced the risk of developing CKD.

Making sure to get enough protein may be especially important for older adults. Some research suggests that older adults who get more than the protein RDA (aiming for 1 to 1.2 grams per kilogram of body weight) may be better able to maintain a healthy body weight, preserve muscle mass, and stay independent as they age. Emerging evidence suggests spreading your protein intake more evenly throughout the day may be especially helpful in

**SMART SHIFT**

## Move Some Protein to Breakfast

Spreading your protein throughout the day helps you maintain—or build—lean muscle. It also helps you feel satisfied longer between meals. People often eat an extra-large serving of protein at dinner, while the protein at breakfast often falls short. Try reducing portions of animal protein at dinner to around 3 ounces (about the size of a deck of cards) and including more protein at breakfast. Each of the low-fuss breakfast ideas below provides at least 20 grams of protein—just add your favorite fruits and veggies.

- 1 cup Greek yogurt and a granola bar (with at least 3 grams of protein)
- ½ cup cottage cheese with ¼ cup nuts and fresh or dried fruit
- 2 ounces of last night's dinner protein on a large slice of whole-grain toast
- ¾ cup dry oats cooked with 1½ cups nonfat milk
- 2 tablespoons nut butter spread on a small whole-grain tortilla wrapped around a banana or apple slices
- 2 eggs (any style) and 1 oz (1 slice) cheese
- 2 eggs in a small whole-grain tortilla, sprinkled with 2 tablespoons grated cheese
- ½ cup quinoa cooked in 1 cup milk, with ¼ cup chopped nuts
- 1 whole-grain English muffin with 1 egg and 2 slices deli turkey
- ½ cup dry oats cooked in 1 cup milk, with 1 tablespoon peanut butter stirred in before eating
- 1 tablespoon peanut butter on a banana, with 1 cupounce eq kefir on the side
- 2 tablespoons peanut butter on a whole-grain English muffin sprinkled with sunflower seeds, and 8 ounces of milk, soymilk, kefir, or regular yogurt
- ¼ cup black beans mixed with 2 tablespoons salsa and spread on a small whole-grain tortilla, topped with ½ cup crumbled tofu or an egg and a sprinkle of shredded cheese

## What Counts as an Ounce-Equivalent of Protein

Here are a few examples of what counts as a 1-ounce equivalent of protein, according to the USDA. Learn more at ChooseMyPlate.gov.

| PROTEIN | AMOUNT EQUIVALENT TO 1 OUNCE OF PROTEIN | COMMON SERVING, IN OUNCE-EQUIVALENTS (OZ-EQ) OF PROTEIN | | |
|---|---|---|---|---|
| Beef, lamb, pork | • 1 oz cooked beef, lamb, or pork | • 1 small steak = 3½ to 4 oz-eq<br>• 1 small lean hamburger = 2 to 3 oz-eq | | |
| Poultry | • 1 oz cooked chicken or turkey without the skin | • 1 small chicken breast half = 3 oz-eq | | |
| Fish/ Shellfish | • 1 oz cooked fish or shellfish | • 1 can of tuna, drained = 3 to 4 oz-eq<br>• 1 salmon steak = 4 to 6 oz-eq | | • 1 small trout = 3 oz-eq |
| Eggs | • 1 egg | • 2 eggs = 2 oz-eq | • 3 egg whites = 3 oz-eq | • 3 egg yolks = 1 oz-eq |
| Nuts and seeds | • ½ oz nuts (12 almonds, 24 pistachios, 7 walnut halves)<br>• ½ oz pumpkin, sunflower, or other seeds<br>• 1 Tbsp peanut or almond butter | • 1 oz nuts or seeds = 2 oz-eq | | |
| Beans and peas | • ¼ cup cooked beans (such as black, kidney, white, pinto)<br>• ¼ cup cooked peas (such as chickpeas, lentils, split peas)<br>• ¼ cup tofu (about 2 oz)<br>• 1 oz tempeh, cooked<br>• ¼ cup roasted soybeans<br>• 2 Tbsp hummus | • 1 cup split pea soup = 2 OE<br>• 1 cup lentil soup = 2 OE<br>• 1 cup bean soup = 2 OE<br>• 1 soy or bean burger patty = 2 OE | | |

Source: https://www.choosemyplate.gov/protein-foods

## Protein in Plants

Many plant foods contain a significant amount of protein. Here are some top sources.

| FOOD | PROTEIN (G) |
|---|---|
| **Soy Foods** | |
| Edamame (green soybeans), ½ cup shelled | 10 |
| Soymilk, 1 cup | 8 |
| Soynuts, ¼ cup | 10 |
| Tempeh, ½ cup | 16 |
| Tofu, ½ cup | 10 |
| **Legumes (cooked)** | |
| Black beans, ½ cup | 8 |
| Chickpeas (garbanzos), ½ cup | 8 |
| Lentils, ½ cup | 9 |
| Pinto beans, ½ cup | 8 |
| Kidney beans, ½ cup | 8 |
| **Seeds** | |
| Hemp seeds, ¼ cup | 12 |
| Pumpkin seeds, ¼ cup | 9 |
| Sunflower seeds, ¼ cup | 6 |
| **Nuts** | |
| Almonds, ¼ cup | 7 |
| Pistachios, ¼ cup | 6 |
| Peanut butter, 2 Tbsp | 7 |
| **Grains (cooked)** | |
| Oatmeal, ½ cup | 3 |
| Quinoa, ½ cup | 4 |
| Teff, ½ cup | 5 |
| Wheat berries, ½ cup | 6 |
| **Vegetables (cooked)** | |
| Asparagus, ½ cup | 2 |
| Peas, ½ cup | 5 |
| Spinach, ½ cup | 3 |

Note: g = grams, Tbsp = tablespoon.
¼ cup nuts or seeds = 1–1.3 ounces.
Source: USDA Food and Nutrient Database

supporting your body's ability to maintain muscle mass as you age.

There are other good reasons to get protein at every meal. Of the three calorie-containing nutrients—protein, carbohydrate, and fat—protein is generally considered the most effective at providing a sense of satiety or fullness. If your breakfast, lunch, or snacks don't seem to have much staying power, they might be low in protein. If you're adding a protein-rich food to a meal, substitute it for something else you'd normally eat (rather than eating it in addition to what you'd typically eat), or you could end up gaining weight.

## Protein and Your Health

There's a lot of focus these days on *how much* protein one should eat, and while some people respond by eating more than they need, thinking that if enough is good, more is better, many others aren't getting enough. When eating with health in mind, it's important to aim for the recommended amount, but it's also important to look at what else your body is getting when you eat those protein-rich foods. The source of protein you choose (such as beef, poultry, seafood, or plants—processed or unprocessed), the cut of meat you buy, and even the way you prepare your meal can all impact your health.

### Source Matters

Animal-based protein sources contribute important nutrients such as zinc, vitamin $B_{12}$, and iron to our diets, but they may also contain unwanted nutrients such as excess saturated fat and sodium. For example, while a ham steak has less saturated fat than the same serving size of a beef steak, it has 20 times more sodium. Wild salmon, on the other hand, has as much protein as the steak and as little saturated fat as the ham, and it's naturally low in sodium. Plus, salmon is an excellent source of heart-healthy omega-3 fats. In fact, all types of seafood are healthful protein sources. The FDA recommends eating 2 to 3 servings, for a total of 8 to 12 ounces, of lower-mercury fish each week.

Plant-based sources of protein, such as nuts and legumes, contribute much-needed nutrients such as fiber, magnesium, vitamin E, and phytochemicals to your diet and are naturally very low in sodium and saturated fat. Soybeans, soy products, and quinoa are particularly good sources of healthful plant protein.

Research backs up the fact that the source of your protein can have a big impact on your health. There has been a particularly strong spotlight on the negative health effects of red and processed meats. They have been implicated in increased risk for cardiovascular disease incidence and death, type 2 diabetes, colon cancer, and even weight gain, and a growing number of studies suggest dietary patterns high in red meat may promote cognitive decline.

Other research generated from the Nurses' Health Study and Health Professionals Follow-Up Study, cohorts that followed 120,000 men and women for more than 20 years, have reported:

- For every 3-ounce serving of unprocessed red meat participants reported eating, the risk of dying from cardiovascular disease increased by 13 percent, and every 1.5 ounces of processed red meat (like bacon, hot dogs, and sausage) increased their risk by 20 percent.
- People who ate the most red and processed meat over the course of the study gained about one extra pound every four years.
- Every additional serving per day of red meat was associated with a 10 percent higher risk of cancer death, and every serving of processed red meat was associated with a 16 percent higher risk.
- A separate study found that every additional serving of red meat increased the risk of developing type 2 diabetes by 12 percent, and processed red meat raised the risk by 32 percent.

In late 2015, the International Agency for Research on Cancer, an independent agency of the World Health Organization

(WHO), released a report recommending that people reduce their intake of processed meats, such as bacon, sausage, hot dogs, jerky, and luncheon meats, because cutting back on them could help reduce the risk of colon cancer. This increased cancer risk may be due to the chemicals added during processing and/or changes in the meat itself due to processing. The report recommended limiting intake of unprocessed red meat, as it is linked with increased cancer risk, as well.

The good news is that cutting back on red meat and replacing red and processed meat with healthy protein sources such as fish, chicken, beans, or nuts seems to reduce health risks. Finally, research has shown that legumes are a healthy alternative to red meat. While eating red meat is associated with weight gain, research found that eating approximately one daily serving of beans, chickpeas, lentils, or peas can help you feel satisfied, which may lead to better weight management.

## Shopping and Cooking

When you do eat red meat, choose the cut of meat carefully. Selecting leaner cuts saves you calories and also helps limit your intake of saturated fat, the type of fat that can raise LDL ("bad") cholesterol and increase heart-disease risk. Look for the words "loin" and "round," which typically signal leaner cuts of meat, such as in "sirloin steak," "top round roast," or "pork tenderloin." Grass-fed beef and bison (available at farmer's markets and some supermarkets) are leaner, too. Besides choosing leaner cuts, trim away any visible fat on the edge of meats before cooking. When preparing poultry, remove the skin either before or after cooking to reduce saturated fat and calories.

When selecting ground meat, choose one that is at least 90 percent lean if it fits your budget. Another option is to blot and/or rinse cooked ground meat with hot water to cut fat. If substituting ground turkey or chicken for ground beef, check the ingredients, since poultry is frequently ground

with the skin. The leanest ground poultry is from pure breast meat.

How you cook your animal protein also matters. Cooking meats at high temperatures using methods such as grilling, broiling, or frying creates potentially cancer-causing compounds, including polycyclic aromatic hydrocarbons and

### The Facts About Mercury in Fish

Fish is a healthful protein source and excellent source of omega-3 fatty acids. Unfortunately, industrial activity, such as coal-fired electricity generation, releases mercury into the air, and that mercury eventually finds its way into bodies of water, where it's consumed by fish. While some fish are high in methyl mercury, most are not. Since big fish eat smaller fish, the higher up on the food chain a fish is, the more contaminated it's likely to be. The current consensus by health professionals is that the health benefits of eating low-mercury fish outweigh the dangers. To help you make informed decisions, the table below indicates likely seafood contamination levels.

| FISH/SHELLFISH | LOW MERCURY | MERCURY COULD ADD UP IF CONSUMED FREQUENTLY* | TOO HIGH IN MERCURY TO EAT REGULARLY** |
|---|:---:|:---:|:---:|
| Anchovies | ✔ | | |
| Atlantic mackerel | ✔ | | |
| Catfish | ✔ | | |
| Clams | ✔ | | |
| Cod | ✔ | | |
| Haddock | | ✔ | |
| Halibut | | ✔ | |
| Herring | ✔ | | |
| Imitation crab (from pollock) | ✔ | | |
| King mackerel | | | ✔ |
| Lobster | | ✔ | ✔ |
| Mahi mahi | | ✔ | |
| Marlin | | | ✔ |
| Mussels | ✔ | | |
| Orange roughy | | | ✔ |
| Oysters | ✔ | | |
| Pollock | ✔ | | |
| Rainbow Trout | ✔ | | |
| Salmon, wild | ✔ | | |
| Sardines | ✔ | | |
| Scallops | ✔ | | |
| Sea Bass | | ✔ | |
| Shark | | | ✔ |
| Shrimp | ✔ | | |
| Swordfish | | | ✔ |
| Tilapia | ✔ | | |
| Tilefish | | | ✔ |
| Tuna, bluefin and bigeye steaks or sushi | | | ✔ |
| Tuna, canned, light and albacore | | ✔ | |

*Pregnant women and children should limit or avoid
**Pregnant women and children should not eat these species.
Source: Environmental Working Group (ewg.org) Consumer Guide to Seafood. Information is also available at the non-profit Environmental Defense Fund's "Seafood Selector," seafood.edf.org.

heterocyclic amines, and can increase the formation of advanced glycation end products (AGEs). AGEs may play a role in the development of diabetic complications like nephropathy, and preliminary data suggest higher levels of AGEs in the brain of individuals with Alzheimer's disease may promote oxidative stress and inflammation. Plant-based foods, such as vegetables, fruits, legumes, and whole grains, contain relatively few AGEs, even after cooking.

Everyone loves a good cookout, so if you're going to grill, soak meat for an hour in an acidic marinade (think lemon juice- or vinegar-based) before cooking and cook meal over a low flame to cut down on the formation of AGEs and carcinogens. Adding herbs, such as oregano, rosemary, or thyme, to the marinade also helps reduce AGEs while boosting flavor.

## A Word About Eggs and Dairy

Eggs and dairy products are excellent protein sources. Eggs were off the menu for many years for people with elevated cholesterol levels because of their high cholesterol content. However, the latest research determined that dietary cholesterol (cholesterol from food) doesn't raise blood cholesterol levels for most people, although the saturated fat found in most high-cholesterol foods might. Other research has shown that egg consumption is not significantly associated with a higher risk of coronary artery disease or type 2 diabetes.

Eggs (and shellfish, such as shrimp) are in the minority of foods high in cholesterol but relatively low in saturated fat, so they are now back on the menu in limited amounts. (For more information on cholesterol, see Chapter 9.) Most people can safely eat up to five to seven eggs per week as part of an overall healthy diet.

Dairy foods provide protein, and they contain other key nutrients that may protect against disease risk. A cup of milk provides eight grams of protein. Greek yogurt has about twice the protein of regular yogurt (around 16 grams per single-serving container). Fermented dairy products, such as yogurt and kefir (keh-FEER), a yogurt drink fermented with yeast in addition to beneficial bacteria, are probiotics that offer many health benefits, not the least of which include supporting

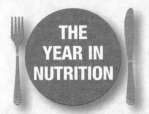

### For Diabetes Prevention, How You Cook Your Meat May Matter

Grilling, broiling, and roasting are popular ways to cook—but are they the healthiest? Recent research out of Harvard University suggests not. In a prospective study that used data collected from 113,561 women from the Nurses' Health Study I and II and 24,679 men from the Health Professional's Follow-up Study, researchers examined the link between open-flame and/or high temperature cooking on risk of developing type 2 DM. All participants were free of diabetes, cardiovascular disease, and cancer at the start of the study and consumed animal foods at at least twice per week.

Over a follow-up period, which ranged from 12 to 16 years, 7,895 individuals developed type 2 diabetes., The researchers found that frequent use of open-flame and high-temperature cooking methods—specifically, broiling and barbecuing chicken, roasting beef, and grilling/barbecuing steak—was associated with higher likelihood of developing diabetes and also with greater weight gain. Adults who ate meat cooked using these techniques on more than 15 occasions per month were at a 28 percent greater risk of developing diabetes compared to those who consumed it less than four times per month.

The authors suggested that their research findings add to the accumulating evidence that cooking meats at high temperatures can produce a number of potentially harmful chemicals that may contribute to the development of diabetes. In their study, the authors found that the intake of one of these chemicals, heterocyclic aromatic amines (HAA), was associated with increased risk of developing diabetes.

One limitation to this study is that the researchers only collected dietary intake information at one timepoint for females and two timepoints for males so their answers may not represent long-term cooking practices. Cutting back on the frequency of eating grilled meats, if you are a fan, may be one modifiable diet factor to consider with respect to reducing diabetes risk.

*Diabetes Care,* March 2018

### Comparing Saturated Fat and Sodium Content in Protein Sources

| 3-OUNCE SERVING | PROTEIN (G) | SATURATED FAT (G) (% DAILY VALUE*) | SODIUM (MG) |
|---|---|---|---|
| Beef (grilled T-bone steak) | 21 | 6.6 (33%) | 53 |
| Pork (ham steak, cured) | 17 | 1.2 (6%) | 1,079 |
| Chicken (boneless skinless breast, roasted) | 26 | 0.9 (4.5%) | 63 |
| Fish (wild Atlantic salmon, broiled) | 22 | 1.1 (5.5%) | 48 |
| Tofu, extra firm, raw** | 9 | 0.5 (2.5%) | 15 |
| Dairy, Greek yogurt, plain, non-fat | 9 | 0.1 (0.5%) | 31 |

*Based on recommendation that saturated fat make up 10% of a 2,000 calorie-a-day diet.
**Nasoya brand Organic Extra Firm Tofu

gut and immune health. Probiotics are live microorganisms that, when administered in adequate amounts, confer a health benefit on the host.

The 2015–2020 *Dietary Guidelines for Americans* recommend fat-free or low-fat (1 percent) milk, which is lower in calories and saturated fat, as well as plain, low-fat yogurt to avoid refined sugars. The *Dietary Guidelines* also state that, although it's okay to eat cheese in moderation, cheese contains more sodium and saturated fat and less potassium, vitamin A, and vitamin D, than milk or yogurt. More than 80 percent of people in the United States fall short of their daily dairy recommendation, which is 3 cups for adults. (For more information on dairy foods, see Chapter 8.)

With about 300 milligrams of calcium per 8 ounces of milk or plain, low-fat yogurt, meeting your daily dairy quota goes a long way toward fulfilling your daily calcium goal. It is recommended that women ages 51 and older consume 1,200 milligrams (mg) of calcium per day, men ages 51 to 70 get 1,000 mg per day, and men ages 71 and older get 1,200 mg per day. Growing evidence suggests it may be best to get most of your calcium from foods, rather than supplements, to help guard against excessive intake of calcium and imbalances in bone nutrients.

To get more dairy in your diet, try using milk in food preparation (to cook oatmeal or to make broth-based soups creamier, for example). If digesting milk is a problem, look for lactose-free options. If a milk substitute is more appealing, make sure it is fortified with calcium and vitamin D, and watch out for added sugars. Also, be aware that, except for soymilk, plant-based "milks" contain little or no protein.

## The Bottom Line

The takeaway is that getting most of your dietary protein from sources such as fish, poultry, beans, nuts, low-fat dairy, and eggs can lower the risk of premature death, cardiovascular disease, diabetes, obesity, and cancer.

If red meat is a staple in your diet, you don't have to give it up. There are many ways to include meat in a healthy dietary pattern.

**THE YEAR IN NUTRITION**

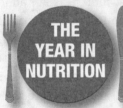

### Have Type 2 Diabetes? Eggs Are Back on the Menu

Although research has shown for some time that there are few links between high egg intake and risk of cardiovascular disease, the jury remained out on whether that was also true for individuals with type 2 diabetes. Results of a recent randomized clinical trial offer good news for egg lovers with diabetes.

The Diabetes and Egg (DIABEGG) Study randomly prescribed a high- or low-egg diet to 140 adult participants with prediabetes or type 2 diabetes. The high-egg plan included two eggs per day at breakfast for six days each week (12 eggs per week), either boiled, poached, or fried in a polyunsaturated cooking oil, such as olive oil. The low-egg group limited eggs to less than two per week, while making up the protein at breakfast with other food sources (lean meat, chicken, fish, legumes, reduced-fat dairy products). After a three-month weight maintenance phase, 128 of the participants continued on their assigned diets, but with reduced calories, in a three-month weight loss phase. The participants were then encouraged to continue with their high- or low-egg prescription for six more months, for a total of 12 months.

Not only was there no significant difference in weight loss between the two groups, there were no significant differences in levels of total cholesterol, LDL ("bad") cholesterol or HDL ("good") cholesterol. Similarly, there were no significant differences in other blood biomarkers that may increase risk of cardiovascular disease. The authors concluded that a high-egg diet is just as safe for people with type 2 diabetes as it is for the general population.

*American Journal of Clinical Nutrition, May 2018*

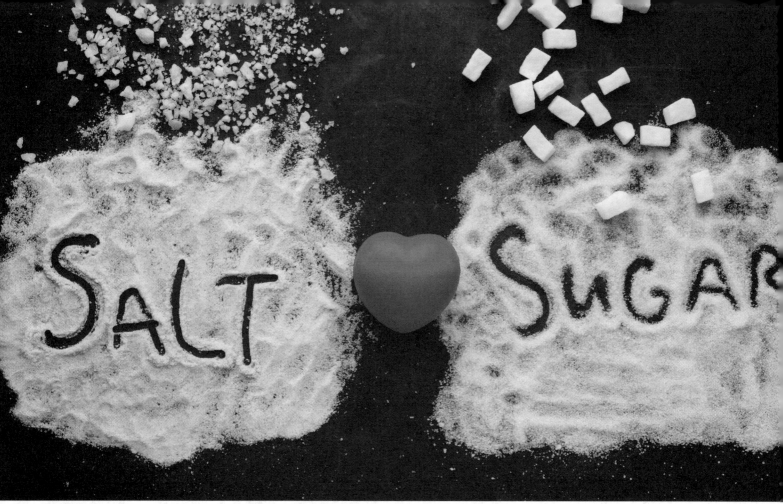

Avoid foods with added sugar or salt.

## 6 Sugar and Salt

**W**hile sugar is one of life's little pleasures and a touch of salt can bring out the flavor in food, consuming too much added sugar and salt (sodium) are both linked to a number of serious health problems. Reducing your intake of added sugars and salt, frequently found in processed foods and other foods prepared outside the home, and allowing your taste buds to appreciate the natural flavors in whole and minimally processed foods, is a key part of creating your personalized healthy eating pattern.

### Spotting Added Sugars in Packaged Foods

Many recommended sugar limits are given in teaspoons, but food labels list sugar in grams. To figure out roughly how many teaspoons of sugar are in a packaged food, divide the number of grams by 4. For example, 20 grams of sugar equals 5 teaspoons.

Added sugars go by many names on package labels, but the body metabolizes them all in essentially the same way. Check ingredient lists for:

- Sugar (white granulated sugar, brown sugar, beet sugar, raw sugar, sugar cane juice)

- Other common names for sugars (cane juice, caramel, corn sweetener, fruit juice/fruit juice concentrate, honey, molasses)

- Nectar (agave nectar, peach nectar, fruit nectar)

- Syrup (corn syrup, high fructose corn syrup, carob syrup, maple syrup, malt syrup)

- Words ending in "–ose" (including sucrose, dextrose, glucose, fructose, maltose, lactose, galactose, saccharose, mannose)

- Foreign or unusual names for sugars (demerara, muscovado, panela/raspadora, panocha/penuche, sweet sorghum, treacle)

### Sugars

When we talk about sugar, what are we talking about, exactly? What we're generally not talking about are the sugars that are naturally present in fruit, vegetables, and milk because these sugars are not a health concern. When you eat whole fruit, for example, your body receives vitamins, minerals, phytochemicals, and fiber along with the sugars. Plus, the amount of sugars you can consume from foods like fruits and vegetables is typically limited, because it would be challenging to eat enough of these foods to get an excessive dose of sugar. Not only does the fiber and other components of whole plant foods fill you up, they may also slow the release of sugars into the bloodstream. On the other hand, foods with added sugars are of concern because they typically provide a large dose of sugar and calories without providing much in the way of fiber or nutrients.

## Added Sugars

Humans long ago figured out how to extract the sugars naturally found in plants (like sugar cane, sugar beets, and corn) and add them to a wide variety of foods. The USDA estimates that, on average, Americans now consume more than 22 teaspoons of these added sugars every day, accounting for approximately 18 percent of the recommended calories for someone consuming 2,000 calories a day. This is nearly double the recommendation of the 2015–2020 *Dietary Guidelines for Americans*, which advise limiting added sugars to less than 10 percent of our daily calories.

The American Heart Association goes even further, recommending that women and children consume no more than six teaspoons (100 calories) of added sugars a day and men no more than nine teaspoons (150 calories). A prospective study of 11,733 U.S. adults found a significant relationship between added sugar consumption and increased risk of death from CVD over 18 years. Those who consumed 17 to 21 percent of their calories from added sugars had a 38 percent higher risk of dying from cardiovascular disease compared with those who consumed only 8 percent of calories from added sugars. Reducing added sugars not only id good for your heart health, but research also suggests it could help reduce the risk of tooth decay, obesity, type 2 diabetes, and some types of cancer in adults. One explanation may be due to AGEs, or Advanced Glycation End products, which were discussed in the previous chapter. A 2017 study found that high sugar intake produces AGEs in the body, and these AGEs may increase inflammation and oxidation in our tissues and organs.

**THE YEAR IN NUTRITION**

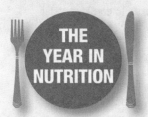

THE YEAR IN NUTRITION

### High Intake of Sugar-Sweetened Beverages May Lead to Fatty Liver

Drinking sugar-sweetened beverages (SSBs) has been tagged as a contributor to weight gain, cardiovascular disease and type 2 diabetes, and now it appears that it may significantly increase the risk of developing non-alcoholic fatty liver disease (NAFLD). NAFLD is an emerging public health concern, largely because it can lead to cirrhosis—the replacement of normal liver tissue with non-living scar tissue—and liver cancer.

A recent systematic review and meta-analysis of six studies, which included a total of 6,326 participants, compared rates of NAFLD among individuals with the highest and lowest intakes of SSBs. The authors found that daily consumption of SSB was associated with a 40 percent greater risk of having NAFLD.

Although the results of this study were limited to data from four cross-sectional studies, the findings are consistent with many previous studies showing a link between SSB intake and increased risk of cardiometabolic diseases (heart disease, stroke, and type 2 diabetes). Liver disease is itself a risk factor for cardiometabolic disease. This may be because not only are SSBs a source of empty calories, but daily intake has been shown to increase fat storage in the liver, muscles, and around the organs, while increasing blood levels of cholesterol and triglycerides. All good reasons to start breaking the SSB habit and drinking more water!

*European Journal of Nutrition,* May 2018

Since excess calories cause weight gain, it has long been thought that sugars increase CVD risk by increasing weight, but a 2014 systematic review and meta-analysis of randomized controlled trials reported CVD risk increased with increased added sugar consumption, regardless of sugar's effect on body weight. In other words, added sugars are bad for your health no matter how thin you are.

## Sugar Is Sugar

In addition to those white crystals in your sugar bowl, added sugars come in many forms, including corn syrup, honey, molasses, maple syrup, brown sugar, agave syrup, fruit juice concentrates, and evaporated cane juice. Most forms of sugars are chemically similar, so switching from one kind of sugar to another won't make a huge difference in terms of your health. The key is to cut back on sweet treats in general. It's estimated that 75 percent of packaged foods sold in the United States contain added sugars, so learning how to spot them is a valuable skill. If you see a sweetener listed as one of the first three ingredients in a packaged food, it likely contains a significant amount of added sugar.

Nearly half of added sugars that people consume are in the form of sugar-sweetened beverages, especially soft drinks, but also fruit drinks, coffee, tea, and sports and energy drinks. Other major sources of added sugars include sweets and snacks, such as candy, ice cream, cookies, granola bars, flavored yogurts, cake, and doughnuts. People also get a significant amount of added sugars from more surprising sources, such as pasta sauces, salad dressings, ketchup, barbecue sauces, breakfast cereals, breads, baked beans, and many other packaged foods.

## Cutting Back

Since added sugars are seemingly everywhere, reducing your dietary intake can seem difficult. The most important thing to remember is that naturally sweet foods are typically healthier than processed sweet foods. Getting more of

**THE YEAR IN NUTRITION**

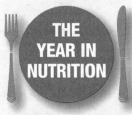

THE YEAR IN NUTRITION

### Consuming More Added Sugars May Increase Risk of Frailty with Age

Diets high in added sugars have been linked to cardiovascular disease and other health conditions, and new research suggests that physical frailty may be another unintended health outcome of consuming too many sugar-sweetened foods and beverages. In a study of 1,973 adults ages 60 or older living in Spain, consuming 36 grams per day or more of added sugars was associated with a 2½ times greater risk of frailty, compared with participants who consumed less than 15 grams per day of added sugars.

To put that in perspective, 36 grams of sugar is within the recommendations set by the *Dietary Guidelines for Americans* and within the American Heart Association recommendations for men (although some people in the high-consumption group did *exceed* 36 grams per day). About one-third of the added sugars consumed by participants came from table sugar, honey or syrup, while two-thirds came from foods like pastries and cookies, which had sugar added during processing. Intake of naturally occurring sugars, such as from fruit or dairy, was not associated with frailty.

Frailty is typically marked by exhaustion, slowness when walking, muscle weakness, unintentional weight loss, and low levels of physical activity. Of these, unintentional weight loss and low levels of physical activity were the markers most associated with greater added sugar intake. While the authors acknowledged that the exact reasons for the association were uncertain, they suggested that high added sugar intake might displace more nutritious sources of calories, including protein and important vitamins and minerals. It's important to continue to eat nutrient-dense foods and incorporate protein foods in our diets as we age, even if we enjoy the occasional sweet dessert!

*American Journal of Clinical Nutrition,* April 2018

## Sugar Surprises

The *2015–2020 Dietary Guidelines for Americans* advise that we limit added sugars to less than 10 percent of our daily calories. For someone eating 2,000 calories a day, that's 50 grams, or about 12 teaspoons (1 teaspoon sugar = approximately 4 g). The American Heart Association recommends only six to nine teaspoons a day. Here's a closer look at how much sugar sneaks into common foods and beverages.

| BEVERAGE ITEM | SERVING | TEASPOONS SUGAR |
|---|---|---|
| Lemon iced tea, sweetened | 16-oz bottle | 13 |
| Energy drink | 16 oz | 12 |
| Cola, regular | 12-oz can | 9 |
| Sports drink | 20-oz bottle | 7½ |
| Meal replacement beverage | 1 bottle | 4 |
| FOOD ITEM | SERVING | TEASPOONS SUGAR |
| Cookies, chocolate sandwich with crème filling | 3 | 8 |
| Pumpkin pie | 1 slice | 6 |
| Raisin bran | 1 cup | 5 |
| Coleslaw | 1 cup | 4.5 |
| Barbecue sauce | 2 tablespoons | 4 |
| Yogurt, low-fat, vanilla | 8 oz | 4 (plus 3½ teaspoons of natural sugar) |
| Doughnut, glazed | 1 medium (3¼ inches) | 3½ |
| Instant oatmeal, flavored | 1 packet | 3 |
| Marinara sauce | ½ cup | 2 |
| Ketchup | 1 tablespoon | 1 |
| Whole-wheat bread | 1 slice | 1 |

your sweet fix from fruits can help you cut back on added sugars: Frozen banana slices puree into an ice cream-like treat that can be flavored however you like (think berries, chocolate, mint, or coffee). Grilled pineapple, fresh strawberries drizzled with balsamic vinegar, and cored, baked apples make simple, delectable desserts. A sweet, juicy orange or peach makes a satisfying (and nutritious) snack when that urge for something sweet hits.

## Sodium

The *2015–2020 Dietary Guidelines for Americans* advise that we consume less than 2,300 milligrams (mg) of sodium, or about 1 teaspoon of salt, per day. Unfortunately, on average, American adults consume approximately 3,500 mg of sodium per day. Typically, as sodium in the diet increases, so does blood pressure. Excess sodium in your bloodstream causes water to be pulled into your blood vessels, increasing blood volume. More blood flowing through your blood vessels increases the pressure on the walls of the vessels—your blood pressure.

Even though most people with high blood pressure have no obvious symptoms, the added pressure can tire out the heart by making it work harder to pump blood through the body, and it also can overstretch blood vessel walls, damaging them. Like a scab that forms on your skin to cover a wound, plaque forms to seal damage in your blood vessels. This plaque can block blood flow, potentially leading to a heart attack or stroke.

That's why sodium also is associated with increased risk of stroke, cardiovascular disease, congestive heart failure, and kidney disease. People ages 51 and older tend to be more affected by the blood-pressure-raising effects of sodium than younger adults.

If you have high blood pressure (hypertension) or prehypertension, the *Dietary Guidelines* recommend reducing your sodium intake to 1,500 mg per day. It can be challenging to reduce sodium to

## SMART SHIFT

### Cut Added Sugars

| INSTEAD OF... | TRY... |
| --- | --- |
| Sugary cereals | Unsweetened cereals with fruit |
| Oatmeal with brown sugar | Steel cut oats with finely chopped date or apple added at the start of cooking, or dried fruit or bananas sprinkled on before eating |
| Sugar-sweetened beverages | Unsweetened drinks like water and unsweetened herbal teas |
| Cookies, cakes, pies | Fresh, frozen, dried, or canned fruit |
| Sugar in recipes | Cut the sugar by a third, or substitute an equal amount of unsweetened applesauce. Extracts like almond, vanilla, orange, or lemon also can add flavor without sugar. |
| Ice cream | Indulge less often; take ½-cup servings; try puréed frozen bananas |
| Fruit-flavored yogurts | Plain yogurt with fresh fruit |
| Sugar, honey or syrup added to beverages or foods | Cut your usual amount in half, then wean down from there |
| Products with a lot of added sugar | Compare labels to find the brand with the lowest added sugar content |

Source: Adapted from American Heart Association

## Salt Versus Sodium

How much sodium does table salt contain? Use this guide.

| | |
| --- | --- |
| ¼ teaspoon salt | = 575 mg sodium |
| ½ teaspoon salt | = 1,150 mg sodium |
| ¾ teaspoon salt | = 1,725 mg sodium |
| 1 teaspoon salt | = 2,300 mg sodium |

Source: American Heart Association

It can take several weeks to get used to a lower sodium intake, but don't give up. Your taste buds will adapt.

recommended limits, but every step you take toward decreasing sodium intake can help in lowering blood pressure. (See Chapter 9 for more on high blood pressure.)

To trim sodium from your diet, you will need to do more than hide the salt shaker—only about 11 percent of our sodium intake comes from salt added during cooking or at the table. Packaged foods and restaurant foods account for the bulk (almost 80 percent) of the sodium in our diets. Reading Nutrition Facts labels can help you scale back on sodium in packaged foods. Restaurant meals often are high in sodium, and it is difficult to determine the amount of sodium in meals when eating out. However, chain restaurants with more than 20 locations now are required to post nutrition information, including sodium content, online, in the restaurant, or both, so be sure to check this information.

Some ways to cut back on sodium include:

- **Prepare more foods at home and from scratch.** Eating out less often can help reduce sodium intake. If you cook whole, unprocessed foods from scratch (as opposed to using pre-packaged foods like flavored rice dishes and canned soups), you'll automatically slash your sodium intake even further.

- **Shop for packaged foods that are lower in sodium.** Foods that have lower sodium content often advertise this on the front of the package. Look for foods marked "low sodium," "no salt added," or "reduced sodium." If you don't like the lower-sodium version, try combining it with the regular version of the food. For example, add some regular canned soup to the low-sodium version and cut back over time as your taste buds adjust.

- **Choose condiments carefully.** Foods like bottled salad dressings, ketchup, mustard, soy sauce, jarred salsa, pickles, and olives are often very high in sodium. Choose lower-sodium versions. "Low-sodium" products contain 140 mg sodium or less per serving. "Reduced sodium" or "less sodium" on a label means the product contains at least 25 percent less sodium than the standard version. Be aware that reduced sodium products may still contain plenty of sodium.

- **Choose poultry that hasn't been injected with sodium solution.** Skip items with terms such as "broth," "saline," or "sodium solution" on the package to avoid unnecessary hidden sodium.

- **Use other seasonings:** Flavoring foods with herbs, spices, garlic, onions, citrus juices, and vinegars can add flavor without salt. When purchasing spice blends, read the label to be certain that salt is not one of the ingredients.

It can take several weeks to get used to a lower sodium intake, but don't give up. Your taste buds will adapt.

Increasing dietary magnesium, calcium, and potassium also are important when it comes to controlling blood pressure. In fact, increasing potassium intake may be as important as reducing sodium intake. The kidneys are responsible for keeping levels of sodium and potassium balanced in the body, so when potassium levels are high, the kidneys excrete more sodium, along with more water. Eating more plant foods is an easy way to increase potassium intake. Beans, sweet potatoes, greens, tomatoes, yogurt, oranges, and bananas are some of the many good sources of this mineral. Many of these potassium-rich foods are part of the DASH dietary pattern, which has been shown to be very effective for lowering blood pressure.

## Herbs and Spices

Herbs and spices are great for flavoring your food without salt. Seasonings generally cost only pennies per serving, and many have potential health benefits. Herbs and spices contain nutrients and phytochemicals that may help lessen inflammation, improve digestion, protect against harmful bacteria, support healthy blood sugar levels, and defend against cancer. Collectively, herbs and spices contain more than 2,000 phytochemicals, many of which act as antioxidants. One study that evaluated the 50 foods highest in antioxidants revealed that the top five were spices (ground cloves, dried oregano, ground ginger, ground cinnamon, and turmeric powder). Examples of common herbs and spices containing anti-inflammatory compounds include chili peppers, black pepper, bay leaves, ginger, marjoram, oregano, rosemary, sage, and thyme. Since you don't typically consume

a lot of these seasonings at one time, the impact they have on your health may not be large, but these tasty plant foods are certainly a simple, healthful way to punch up the flavor of your food without picking up the salt shaker.

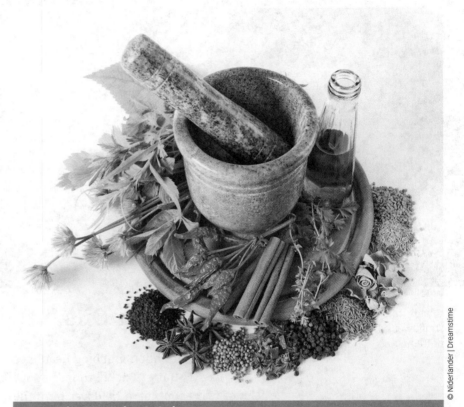

© Niderlander | Dreamstime

### Facts About Herbs & Spices

**Herbs:**

Herbs are obtained from the leaves of plants with woody or non-woody stems.

Examples include: parsley, basil, mint, rosemary, and thyme.

They may be used fresh or dry.

The following amounts of herbs are generally equivalent to each other:

- ¼ to ½ teaspoon ground dried herbs
- 1 teaspoon crumbled dried herbs
- 1 tablespoon finely cut fresh herbs

**Spices:**

Spices are obtained from woody and non-woody plants and come from many different parts of the plant.

Examples include:

- Roots (ginger)
- Flower buds (cloves)
- Flower stigmas (saffron)
- Berries (peppercorns)
- Seeds (cumin)
- Bark (cinnamon)

Spices are typically dried before use.

### General Storage Guidelines*

**Ground spices** (such as ground red pepper): 2 to 3 years
**Whole spices** (such as cinnamon sticks): 3 to 4 years
**Seasoning blends** (such as Italian seasoning): 1 to 2 years
**Herbs** (such as basil leaves): 1 to 3 years
**Extracts** (such as lemon extract): 4 years. Note: Vanilla extract lasts indefinitely.

*If marked with a "best by" date, replace at that time to ensure freshness.

Source: mccormick.com

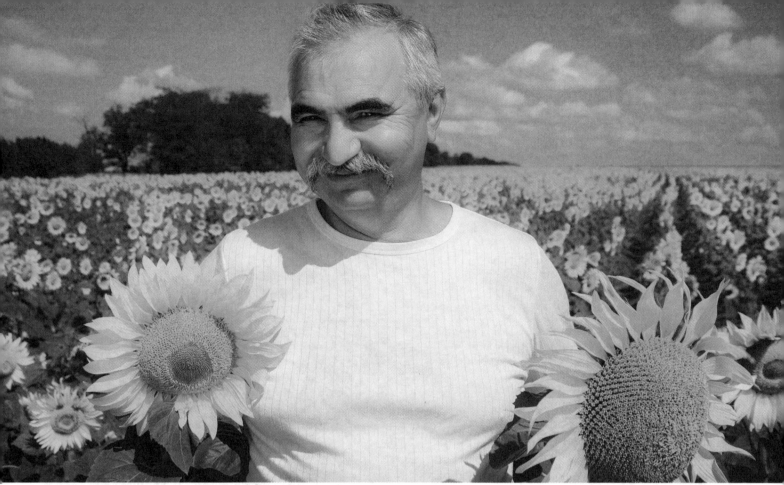

© Oleg Tovkach | Dreamstime

Healthy fats, like the ones in sunflower oils, are important nutrients.

## 7 Fats and Oils

Despite attention-grabbing headlines like "Is Butter Back?" there's still a lot of fear about fat, a holdover from the low-fat era, which peaked in the 1980s and 1990s. But while butter is *not* back, other than in small amounts, fats (also called "fatty acids") perform many essential functions in the body. They are essential for the formation of our cell membranes. They are converted to chemical regulators in the body that affect inflammation, blood clotting, blood-vessel dilation, and more. Including some fat in our meals helps the body absorb fat-soluble nutrients from foods, such as vitamins A, D, E, and K, and disease-fighting phytochemicals such as carotenoids and flavonoids. So, when you have that salad with nutrient-packed dark leafy greens and other veggies, make sure you don't dress it with fat-free dressing.

The 2015–2020 *Dietary Guidelines for Americans* (DGA) advise that a healthy total fat intake can range from 20 to 35 percent of daily calories. Currently, Americans are at the high end of that recommended range, with about 34 percent of calories in the average diet coming from fat. Despite fearing fat, we're eating fat. But are we eating the right fats?

DIETLIFE TIPS

- ◗ **Worry less about total fat—it matters less than the type of fat consumed.** It's fine to get 20 to 35 percent of your daily calories from fats, provided you're choosing the right kinds of fat.

- ◗ **Avoid trans fat.** This dangerous fat is being removed from processed and restaurant-fried foods. Amounts under 0.5 grams are still allowed, so make sure to check ingredient lists for "partially hydrogenated oil," an indicator that a product contains trans fat.

- ◗ **Replace saturated fat.** Cutting back on saturated fat (typical in meats, full-fat dairy, and tropical oils like coconut and palm oil) can reduce your risk of chronic disease, but only if you replace those calories with energy from unsaturated fats, whole grains, and plant proteins—not from refined carbohydrates.

- ◗ **Enjoy healthy unsaturated fats.** Use non-tropical plant oils instead of solid fats, enjoy avocados in moderation, sprinkle nuts and seeds on cereals, salads, and snacks, and eat fatty fish a couple times per week. Just don't go overboard—even healthy fats are high in calories.

A mounting body of evidence shows that it's more important to choose healthier fats than to avoid eating fat altogether. It's also clear that a low-fat diet is not necessarily a healthy one. While many nutritious foods are naturally low in fat, such as vegetables, fruits, whole grains, and legumes, many low-fat foods are not so healthy. Research has found that many packaged foods that carry a low-fat claim are not necessarily nutritious and may be high in added sugar. In keeping with this, the DGA arises that a healthy eating pattern includes oils such as canola, olive, flaxseed, safflower, or sunflower oil, but limits fats associated with increased health risks, such as trans fat and saturated fat.

The DGA recommends consuming:

‣ **No trans fat** (partially hydrogenated oils)

‣ **Less than 10 percent of daily calories from saturated fat** (found primarily in meat, full-fat dairy products, and coconut, palm, and palm kernel oils)

‣ **More foods that contain mono- and polyunsaturated fats** (abundant in non-tropical plant oils such as canola, safflower, sunflower, corn, olive, and soybean oils, as well as nuts, seeds, seafood, and avocados)

The following sections will examine the latest information on these different types of fats and provide a better understanding of dietary fat recommendations.

## Trans Fat

The FDA deems man-made trans fat to be more harmful to cardiovascular health than any other fat, including saturated fat. Artificial trans fat has been shown to raise triglyceride and LDL (bad) cholesterol levels, lower HDL (good) cholesterol levels, promote inflammation, and worsen insulin resistance.

Small amounts of trans fat may occur naturally in some milk and meat products, but a much larger concern is artificial trans fat, created by an industrial process that adds hydrogen to liquid vegetable oils to make them more solid. These "hydrogenated oils" and "partially hydrogenated oils" were widely used in processed foods and for deep-frying in fast-food outlets and restaurants before the FDA determined they were not safe. Trans fats were used to extend the shelf life of processed foods and gave them

---

### Trim Trans Fat from Your Diet

The American Heart Association offers the following advice for avoiding trans fat:

- Look for "0 g trans fat" on the Nutrition Facts label and no hydrogenated or partially hydrogenated oils in the ingredients list.

- Doughnuts, cookies, crackers, muffins, pies, and cakes are examples of foods that may contain trans fat. Limit how frequently you eat them.

- Limit commercially fried foods and baked goods made with shortening or partially hydrogenated vegetable oils.

- Use naturally occurring, non-hydrogenated plant oils such as olive, avocado, canola, safflower, or sunflower oil most often.

- If you're going to purchase processed foods, look for items made with non-hydrogenated oil rather than partially hydrogenated or hydrogenated vegetable oils or saturated fat.

- Use soft margarine rather than stick margarine.

- Eat a dietary pattern that emphasizes whole and minimally processed foods; avoid highly processed, packaged foods.

---

**THE YEAR IN NUTRITION**

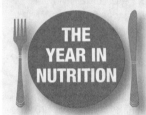

### Smart Snacking May Improve Cholesterol Levels

Could choosing almonds for a snack instead of something high in refined carbohydrates help improve your HDL ("good") cholesterol? A study of 48 middle-aged adults with high cholesterol were randomly assigned to eat 43 unsalted whole almonds (1.5 ounces) or a banana muffin (control) for six weeks. Both snacks had similar calories, but the almond snack was lower in carbohydrates and higher in total fat than the muffin snack. The rest of the participants' diets were identical and designed to be cholesterol-lowering, limiting saturated fat to 8 percent of total calories. Including the snacks, the "almond diet" was higher in total fat (32 vs. 26 percent for the control diet) and lower in carbohydrates (51 vs. 58 percent).

At the start of the study, the participants had high LDL ("bad") cholesterol and normal HDL cholesterol. They followed one assigned diet for six weeks followed by another diet for six weeks, in what is called a cross-over trial. In participants with a body mass index (BMI) in the normal range, the almond diet improved HDL cholesterol and had favorable effects on HDL particle size and function. The same results, however, were not observed in overweight or obese study participants. While this study is of short duration and among a relatively small number of subjects, the data suggests that substitution of nuts for a refined grain snack may improve HDL cholesterol in normal weight adults with high cholesterol. Keep in mind when making changes to your diet to substitute rather than add a new food to your diet. Incorporating nuts into your diet is one dietary strategy for improving your lipid profile!

*The Journal of Nutrition, August 2017*

a desirable taste and texture. For example, trans fats helped to keep frozen pizza crusts flaky. The FDA required that trans fat be removed from foods by June 2018 (unless the manufacturer received a waiver from the FDA to allow its use in a specific product), although foods produced before the deadline can be sold until they run out.

Per labeling rules, if a food contains less than 0.5 grams of trans fat per serving, the amount of trans fat can be rounded down to 0 on the Nutrition Facts label. Thus, if you eat more than the recommended serving size of a food, you could be ingesting a significant amount of trans fat. This means you must check the ingredient list; if "partially hydrogenated oil" appears, the product contains trans fat. Pay special attention to fried foods and baked goods as well as frostings, margarines, and other spreads made by solidifying oils. Even small amounts of trans fat are harmful to health and should be avoided when possible.

## The Coconut Oil Conundrum

Is coconut oil a superfood or a dangerous choice for replacing other fats? While 72 percent of Americans in a 2016 survey thought coconut oil was healthy, only 37 percent of dietitians agreed. The source of this disagreement is the complex science surrounding fatty acid metabolism.

Fatty acids are made up of chains of carbon atoms. These chains can vary in length (short, medium, or long), and the carbons can be saturated with hydrogen atoms or unsaturated. These variables determine how the chains are absorbed, transported, and used by the body. The "fats" we eat, such as olive oil, soybean oil, butter, or coconut oil, are each made up of a different mixture of these various types of fatty acids.

Coconut oil has a large proportion of medium-chain fatty acids (MCFA) compared to other fats and oils used for cooking. MCFAs with a length of eight or 10 carbons are easily absorbed and are converted to fuel very efficiently. For this reason, they have been associated with some health benefits. However, the MCFAs in coconut oil are a bit longer, mostly 12 carbons long. In some ways, they behave like eight- or 10-carbon chains, but in other ways, they are more like long-chain fatty acids, which are used less efficiently by our bodies. Coconut oil also is much higher in saturated fat than other plant oils, such as olive and canola oils. Most experts agree that consuming saturated fatty acids is bad for your health.

The bottom line: Claims that consuming coconut oil helps with weight loss, reduces cardiovascular disease or dementia risk, and prevents or treats diabetes are not backed up by any strong scientific evidence. We know this tropical oil is a rich source of saturated fats, which all major policy organizations recommend you avoid. Until scientists have a better understanding of what those 12-carbon chains do in your body, it's best to use plant oils that are higher in unsaturated fatty acids (such as olive and canola oils) and save coconut oil for cooking the occasional tropics-inspired dish that benefits from its nutty flavor.

## What Is Saturated Fat?

Fatty acids are chains of carbon atoms with hydrogen atoms attached to them. If the carbons are full, there is no room for any more hydrogen atoms and the fat is called *saturated*. Meat, full-fat dairy products, tropical oils such as coconut, palm, and palm kernel oil, and products made with these ingredients, are major sources of saturated fat. When isolated, saturated fats are solid at room temperature, whereas unsaturated fats (like olive, avocado, canola, or other plant oils) are liquid. The American Heart Association states that consuming saturated fat is proven to raise your LDL ("bad") cholesterol and put you at higher risk for heart disease.

The DGA recommends consuming no more than 10 percent of your daily calories from saturated fat (that's about 20 grams for someone eating 2,000 calories a day). The American Heart Association advises restricting intake of saturated fat further, to no more than 5 to 6 percent of daily calories.

In recent years, some headlines touted the findings of research studies that reportedly found no health benefits associated with reducing total and/or saturated fat intake. Yet, recent data from a large observational study reinforced the idea that higher dietary intake of saturated fat is indeed associated with an increased risk of coronary heart disease. In addition, other observational studies also have linked higher intakes of saturated fat with increased risk for diabetes.

Importantly, research indicates that it's important to consider what replaces saturated fat in the diet. Replacing saturated fat with refined carbohydrate foods like "low-fat" cookies, cakes, and crackers could also increase your heart disease risk. In other words, if you want to see health benefits associated with lowering saturated fat intake, don't replace foods high in saturated fat with refined carbohydrate foods. Instead, choose foods that are sources of unsaturated fats. For example, make the switch to olive or other plant oils instead of butter or other solid fats in cooking, eat more fish in place of red meat, and use vegetable-oil based dressings rather than creamy choices. When snacking, choose veggies and a bean-based dip like hummus instead of chips and a creamy dip, pick a fruit-and-nut bar instead of a candy bar, have whole-grain toast with nut butter instead of a pastry. Replacing saturated fats with whole grains or plant proteins has also been linked to reduced heart-disease risk. Data analysis based on two recent large observational studies on fat intake and heart disease suggest that replacing even 1 percent of your daily calories from saturated fat with the same number of calories from either unsaturated fats, whole grains, or plant proteins could reduce heart disease risk by 6 to 12 percent.

Keep in mind that most foods contain a mixture of different types of fatty acids, some saturated and some unsaturated. When cooking and dressing your foods, it's recommended you choose plant oils, which are high in mono- and/or polyunsaturated fats, while low in saturated fats.

## Unsaturated Fats

Unsaturated fats are found in foods such as plant oils, nuts, seeds, and fish. There are two types of unsaturated fatty acids, monounsaturated and polyunsaturated, both of which have health benefits.

Observational studies indicate that a lower intake of saturated fat, coupled with a higher intake of mono- or polyunsaturated fats, is associated with lower rates of CVD. Research using statistical models indicates that swapping out just 5 percent of calories from saturated fat for equivalent amounts of poly- or monounsaturated fats reduced coronary heart-disease risk by 25 percent in men and 15 percent in women.

According to an American Heart Association Presidential Advisory issued in June 2017, participants in randomized, controlled trials who replaced saturated fat with polyunsaturated vegetable oil reduced their risk of cardiovascular disease by approximately 30 percent. This is similar to the improvement achieved by taking cholesterol-lowering statin drugs.

Replacing some of the carbohydrates in your diet with unsaturated fats also can have favorable effects on your diabetes risk. A systematic review and meta-analysis of data from 24 randomized controlled trials (with a total of 1,460 participants who had type 2 diabetes) found that when compared to high-carbohydrate diets, diets high in monounsaturated fats from plant sources like olive oil, avocados, and nuts were associated with lower fasting blood sugar as well as lower triglycerides, blood pressure, and body weight. Levels of HDL ("good") cholesterol also were higher. When compared with a diet high in polyunsaturated fats, a high-monounsaturated fat diet was

### Comparing Fatty Acid Content of Fats and Oils

All fats and oils are a mixture of fatty acids, which include three main types: monounsaturated, polyunsaturated (including omega-3 and omega-6), and saturated.

You may hear people refer to olive oil as a monounsaturated fat, since it contains significantly more monounsaturated fatty acids than most other oils. In reality, however, it is a combination of fatty acids, just like any other fat. This graph compares the percentages of different fatty acids in common fats and oils.

| FAT SOURCE | MONO | POLY | SAT |
|---|---|---|---|
| Avocado oil | 71% | 13% | 16% |
| Butter | 30% | 4% | 66% |
| Canola oil | 64% | 29% | 7% |
| Coconut oil | 6% | 2% | 92% |
| Corn oil | 25% | 62% | 13% |
| Hazelnut oil | 81% | 11% | 8% |
| Lard | 47% | 12% | 41% |
| Olive oil | 77% | 9% | 14% |
| Palm oil | 39% | 10% | 51% |
| Palm kernel oil | 12% | 2% | 86% |
| Peanut oil | 48% | 34% | 18% |
| Safflower oil | 13% | 78% | 9% |
| Sunflower oil | 20% | 69% | 11% |
| Soybean oil | 24% | 61% | 15% |

Poly = polyunsaturated fatty acids; Mono = monounsaturated fatty acids; Sat = saturated fatty acids

### SMART SHIFT — Fats for Better Health

To replace saturated fat with unsaturated fats:

| INSTEAD OF... | CHOOSE... |
|---|---|
| Butter or lard | Plant-based spreads or oils (olive, avocado, corn, canola, or soybean) |
| Red meat | Fish |
| Whole milk | Low- or nonfat milk |
| Meat chili | Bean chili |
| Ground meat | Ground chicken or turkey breast, meatless crumbles, or crumbled firm tofu sautéed in vegetable oil |
| Bacon on salad | Pumpkin seeds or walnuts on salad |
| Buttered popcorn | Popcorn air-popped or prepared with vegetable oil |
| Coconut "milk" | Fortified soy or almond "milk" |
| Chocolate-flavored hazelnut spread | Unsweetened peanut butter or almond butter |
| Candy bar | Dried fruit/nut bar |
| Meat lasagna | Vegetable lasagna |
| Two slices of pizza | One slice (with veggie topping) and a side salad with vinaigrette |
| Beef tacos | Fish tacos |

Source: adapted from *Tufts Health & Nutrition Letter*, May 2017

associated with lower blood glucose, but no other significant differences.

## Omega-3 and Omega-6 Fatty Acids

The two most commonly studied types of polyunsaturated fatty acids are omega-3s and omega-6s. These are both essential fatty acids, which means they

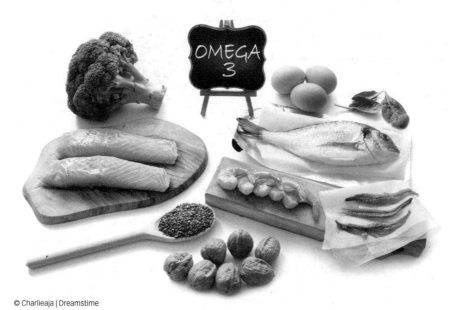

© Charlieaja | Dreamstime

are necessary for health but cannot be manufactured by the body and must be obtained from food. Omega-3 fatty acids have been associated with health benefits such as improving cardiovascular health, protecting cognitive function, and promoting longevity. An analysis of 19 studies involving 45,637 participants in 16 countries found that higher blood levels of omega-3s (from seafood and plants) were associated with lower risk of dying from heart attacks. People with the highest blood levels of omega-3s weren't less likely to have a heart attack compared with people with the lowest levels, but they had about a 25 percent lower risk of *dying* from a heart attack.

Fish is the major food source of the well-studied, health-promoting omega-3 fatty acids eicosapentaenoic acid (EPA) and docosahexaenoic acid (DHA). All fish and seafood contain some omega-3s. The highest levels are found in fatty fish, including salmon, trout, anchovies, sardines, and herring. Most policy organizations, including the USDA, recommend consuming at least

---

**THE YEAR IN NUTRITION**

### Foods Rich in Unsaturated Fats

Foods high in mono- and polyunsaturated fats include:

- **Liquid plant oils** such as olive, avocado, peanut, canola, flaxseed, sunflower, corn, and soybean oils and spreads made from these oils

- **Avocados and olives**

- **Nuts** such as walnuts, almonds, hazelnuts, cashews, pistachios, peanuts, and pecans

- **Seeds** such as pumpkin, flax, chia, sunflower, and sesame seeds

- **Fish,** particularly fatty fish such as salmon, mackerel, herring, lake trout, sardines, and albacore tuna

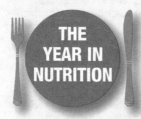

THE YEAR IN NUTRITION

### Higher Omega-3 Intake May Reduce Glaucoma Risk

Glaucoma is the leading cause of irreversible blindness in both eyes. The biggest known risk factors for developing this condition are family history of glaucoma, being female or African American, and getting older. None of those risk factors are modifiable, so there is significant interest in what risk factors can be modified. Currently, there are medical and surgical options for reducing pressure within the eye, which is another risk factor for glaucoma. What about diet though?

Researchers looked at data from 3,865 participants in the National Health and Nutrition Examination Survey (NHANES), focusing on participants age 40 and older who had undergone an eye examination to detect glaucoma. Because previous clinical research found that people with glaucoma had lower blood levels of the omega-3 fatty acids eicosapentaenoic acid (EPA) and docosahexaenoic acid (DHA), this study aimed to look at associations between both omega-3 and omega-6 fatty acids—both of which are polyunsaturated fatty acids (PUFAs)—and the risk of glaucoma.

In this cross-sectional study, increased consumption of EPA and DHA were associated with lower risk of glaucoma, but higher intake of other types of polyunsaturated fats was associated with increased risk. The benefits of EPA and DHA may be due to improved blood flow in the eye and the anti-inflammatory effects of omega-3s, which are primarily found in fatty fish like salmon and sardines. Interestingly, higher total consumption of PUFAs was higher in people who developed glaucoma, but, as noted by the authors, this observation needs to be further investigated with clinical studies.

*JAMA Ophthalmology,* February 2018

two servings of fatty fish per week. The omega-3s found in seeds, nuts, and their oils are called lpha-linolenic acid (ALA). Your body converts some, but not all, of the ALA you consume into EPA and DHA. While ALA has been shown to have its own health benefits, it's not a replacement for EPA and DHA.

Omega-6 fatty acids also are found in vegetable oils, seeds, and nuts. You may have heard that you should avoid omega-6 fats because they increase disease-producing inflammation. However, many of the studies backing this claim were performed on animals, and controlled studies in which people were fed oil rich in omega-6 fats failed to show an increase in markers of inflammation. In fact, polyunsaturated fatty acids are precursors to a family of compounds (eicosanoids) that help mediate and regulate inflammation, so they actually may have anti-inflammatory effects.

## Nuts and Seeds

Nuts and seeds are rich in healthy monounsaturated and polyunsaturated fatty acids and provide vitamin E, antioxidants, and other phytochemicals. Studies suggest that eating one ounce (about ¼ cup) of nuts daily might help improve mood, control hunger, boost longevity, reduce diabetes risk, and help fight heart disease and stroke. A recent review of 61 controlled trials found that people who included about ¼ cup of tree nuts (walnuts, pistachios, macadamia nuts, pecans, cashews, almonds, hazelnuts, and Brazil nuts) in their daily diets had reduced total cholesterol, unhealthy LDL cholesterol, and triglycerides. Nuts are high in fat, but a high proportion of that fat is polyunsaturated. Be aware, however, that nuts, like all fat-rich foods, are high in calories (approximately 160 to 200 calories per ounce), so limit the total amount you eat to a handful and replace other foods with nuts rather than merely adding them to your diet. For example, instead of chips, snack on nuts, and top your salad with chopped nuts rather than croutons.

Like nuts, seeds have some impressive nutrition credentials. Chia and sesame seeds, for example, are particularly good sources of calcium, with 1-ounce servings providing 179 and 277 milligrams, respectively. Flax and chia seeds are rich in ALA, the plant version of healthy omega-3 fats. A 1-ounce serving of sunflower seeds provides more than half the recommended dietary allowance for vitamin E. Sunflower-seed butter tastes delicious and makes a great substitute for nut butters for those with nut allergies.

**THE YEAR IN NUTRITION**

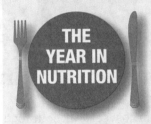

### For Diabetes Risk, Not All Fats Are Created Equal

When you think of foods that might increase risk of developing type 2 diabetes, you probably think of sugar and other carbohydrates, but the types of dietary fat you choose may also play a role, according to recent research out of Spain.

Researchers followed 3,349 participants from the PREDIMED for an average of 4.3 years to look for associations between intake of total fat and specific types of fat and new cases of type 2 diabetes. While all PREDIMED participants were at high risk of developing cardiovascular disease, participants included in this analysis did not have type 2 diabetes when enrolled in the study. About one-third of the participants were assigned to eat a Mediterranean diet enriched with extra virgin olive oil, one-third ate a Mediterranean diet enriched with nuts, and the final third served as a control group. Over a follow-up period of 4.3 years, 266 participants developed type 2 diabetes.

The study results suggested that greater intake of saturated fats, particularly animal fats, were associated with an increased risk of developing type 2 diabetes. When the authors looked closer at specific foods, they found that cheese and butter were associated with increased risk, while full-fat yogurt was associated with a decreased risk. Foods like eggs, whole fluid milk, and red meat appeared to neither increase nor decrease risk of developing diabetes. Overall, the results of this study support current dietary recommendations to choose plant-based fats most of the time.

*American Journal of Clinical Nutrition*, March 2017

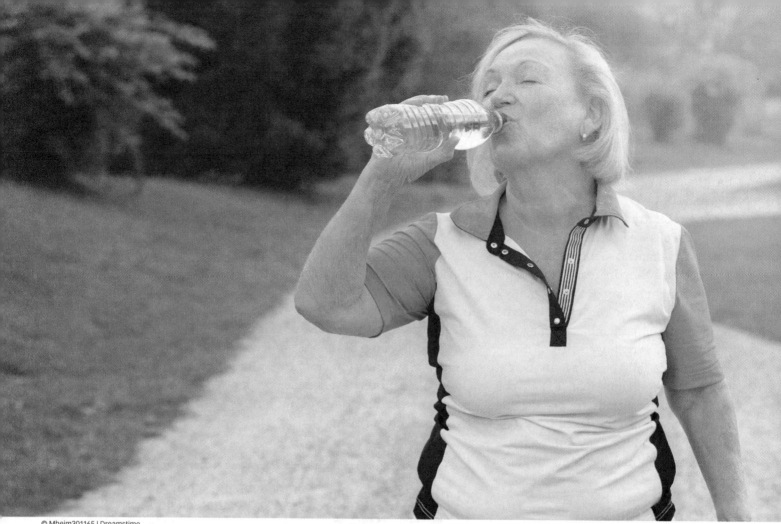

© Mheim301165 | Dreamstime

Water is a biological necessity, but you don't have to just drink it. Fruits, vegetables, and other foods contain water that adds to our daily intake.

## 8 Beverages: Staying Hydrated

Your body can go weeks without food, albeit with the detrimental side effects of a lowered metabolism and loss of lean muscle, but you can only live a few days without fluids. At least 60 percent of the adult body is made of water, and every living cell needs it to function. Water transports nutrients, lubricates your joints and body tissues, facilitates digestion, allows your kidneys to remove waste products from your body in urine, maintains blood pressure and circulation, and helps preserve normal body temperature through sweating.

So how much water is enough? The Dietary Reference Intakes (DRI) specify that the adequate intake level for fluids is 12 cups (95 ounces) per day for women and 16 cups (130 ounces) per day for men, but not all of that comes from what you drink.

One of many reasons to eat lots of fruits and vegetables is that they are water-rich. Foods like soup and cooked cereal also will help you meet your water quota. It's estimated that people get 20 to 30 percent of their water from food. That still requires that women drink 8 to 10 cups per day and that men drink 11 to 13 cups per day to meet the DRI, although individual needs vary. Older adults tend to have a reduced sense of thirst and lower fluid reserves in their body, and they may be taking medications such as diuretics that increase water loss, so they may need to pay more attention to their fluid intake to avoid becoming dehydrated. Sweating (from exercise or heat) also increases fluid needs.

### What to Drink

Water is the best choice for keeping you hydrated, but unflavored milk (or calcium-fortified unsweetened milk substitutes), tea, and coffee (hold the sugar, syrups, and whipped cream) also are good choices. Contrary to myth, if you are a regular coffee drinker, you don't need to drink an extra glass of water for every cup of coffee. If you drink coffee habitually, you develop a tolerance for the potential diuretic effects of caffeine.

Keep in mind that even though 100-percent fruit juices may be hydrating, and contain only natural fruit sugars, drinking large volumes may cause spikes in blood sugar and, if providing excess calories, may lead to weight gain. Furthermore, liquid calories, such as from orange juice, may not provide as much satiety (sense of fullness) as calories from solid foods, such as from a whole orange. Limit your juice consumption to 8 ounces per day or less.

## Water

A cool glass of water is calorie-free, readily available, and refreshing. If you find the taste of water boring, punch up the flavor a bit. Fill a pitcher with water and add a squeeze of lemon, lime, or orange juice, a few crushed berries, slices of cucumber or ginger root, or fresh mint leaves.

Beyond keeping you hydrated, drinking more water may help you lose weight and make healthier food choices. Researchers at the University of Illinois at Urbana-Champaign examined the dietary habits of more than 18,300 U.S. adults over seven years and found that those who increased their water consumption by only one or two cups per day decreased their calorie intake as well as their consumption of saturated fat, sugar, sodium, and cholesterol. Adults who made this small change reduced their total energy intake by 68 to 205 calories per day, and sodium intake dropped by 78 to 235 milligrams. Even increasing the percentage of fluids coming from water by only 1 percent improved the overall diet. It doesn't matter if you get your water from the tap, a water cooler, a drinking fountain, or a bottle, choosing water over other beverages is a good choice for your health.

## Milk

The 2015–2020 *Dietary Guidelines for Americans* recommend adults consume 3 cups per day of dairy products such as milk and yogurt. More than 80 percent of people in the United States fall short of this recommendation. Milk is an excellent source of vitamins and minerals that Americans tend to fall short on. These vitamins and minerals include calcium, potassium, magnesium, and, if fortified, vitamins A and D. Milk also supplies protein, riboflavin

### Dehydration

Dehydration happens when you don't take in enough fluid or you lose too much fluid. Some signs of mild to moderate dehydration include thirst, a dry mouth, decreased urination, dark yellow urine, dry skin, headache, and/or muscle weakness or cramps. It may also contribute to constipation. Dehydration is most commonly caused by not adequately replacing fluids lost from diarrhea, vomiting, increased urination with diabetes, and sweating.

Thirst is the body's way of prompting us to drink fluids to maintain adequate hydration levels. When your body loses more water than you take in, it triggers thirst. Older adults are at greater risk of dehydration from small losses of water because the amount of water in the body decreases by about 15 percent between the ages of 20 and 80. Older adults also tend not to feel as thirsty, so they typically become more dehydrated before thirst is triggered compared to a younger person.

Water is usually the best way to stay hydrated. Since water leaves the body as sweat, the risk of dehydration increases with intense physical activity if you don't drink enough fluids during workouts to make up for the fluid losses. Be sure to start exercise—especially during hot weather—adequately hydrated, and drink regularly to maintain hydration levels.

Signs of severe dehydration include dizziness or lightheadedness, unusual fatigue or sleepiness, maple syrup-colored urine, very dry skin, sunken eyes, unusually rapid heartbeat, and low systolic (top number) blood pressure (100 mmHg or less). Severe dehydration can contribute to many common health concerns, including falls, urinary tract infections, and kidney stones.

### Nutrients in Milk and Milk Substitutes (1 cup is 8 fl oz)

| | PROTEIN (G) | CALCIUM* (MG) | TOTAL FAT (G) | SAT FAT (G) | CALORIES |
|---|---|---|---|---|---|
| Dairy, 1% fat milk * | 8 | 300 | 2.5 | 1.5 | 99 |
| Soy milk, fortified, unsweetened * | 7 | 300 | 4 | 0.5 | 79 |
| Hemp milk, fortified, unsweetened | 3 | 283 | 4.5 | 0 | 60 |
| Almond milk, fortified, unsweetened * | 1.0 | 482 | 2.5 | 0 | 39 |
| Coconut milk, fortified, unsweetened | 1 | 451 | 5 | 5 | 74 |
| Rice milk, fortified, unsweetened * | 0 | 283 | 2 | 0 | 113 |

g = grams; mg = milligrams; sat fat = saturated fat.
*Values are for products fortified with calcium and vitamin D and may vary by brand.
Source: USDA Food Composition Databases ndb.nal.usda.gov/ndb

| What Counts as a Cup of Dairy | |
|---|---|
| It is recommended that adults consume three cups of dairy or dairy-equivalent a day. Here are a few examples of what counts as 1 cup of dairy, in the MyPlate Dairy Group. Learn more at ChooseMyPlate.gov. | |
| **FOOD** | **AMOUNT EQUIVALENT TO 1 CUP (8 FLUID OUNCES)** |
| Milk | • 1 cup |
| Yogurt | • 1 cup |
| Cheese | • 1½ oz hard cheese, such as cheddar, Parmesan, Swiss, gouda<br>• ⅓ cup shredded cheese<br>• 2 oz processed American cheese<br>• ½ cup ricotta cheese<br>• 2 cups cottage cheese |
| Soymilk | • 1 cup |
| Evaporated milk | • ½ cup |

(vitamin B2), vitamin B12, choline, zinc, and selenium. Many of these nutrients, most notably calcium, vitamin D, and magnesium, are essential for healthy bones. Dairy products have earned their place in healthy dietary patterns for several reasons beyond their vitamin and mineral content. Studies have linked regular consumption of dairy products to lower blood pressure in adults and a reduced risk of cardiovascular disease, stroke, type 2 diabetes, and weight gain.

There are numerous milk alternatives in grocery stores, but many are not nutritionally equivalent to milk, especially if they're not fortified with calcium and vitamin D. Typically, fortified soymilk is nutritionally similar to cow's milk. Always read labels: Many plant-based milk substitutes are low in protein, and some are sweetened, which adds to their calories and to your daily added sugar total.

## Coffee and Tea
Coffee and tea are two of the most commonly consumed beverages around the world. Both beverages are frequent subjects of research studies, many of which indicate that these beverages deliver health benefits.

According to the 2015–2020 *Dietary Guidelines for Americans,* moderate coffee drinking (three to five 8-ounce cups per day for healthy adults; two cups a day if pregnant) can be part of a healthy dietary pattern. Coffee is rich in many beneficial compounds, such as chlorogenic acids and other polyphenols, magnesium, and antioxidant lignans. Such compounds may contribute to the benefits associated with coffee drinking, including lower risks of stroke, arterial plaque (atherosclerosis), type 2 diabetes, depression, Parkinson's disease, and Alzheimer's disease, as well as improved longevity. Research from the Multiethnic Cohort (MEC) study, a large, population-based study that began in the 1990s, found that compared with drinking no coffee, drinking at least one cup per day of caffeinated or decaffeinated coffee was associated with lower risk of death from all causes, and drinking two or more cups appeared to offer even more protection. The findings applied to both men and women of all ages and different racial/ethnic groups.

On a cautionary note, however, skip the French press and coffee percolator. Instead, brew your coffee using a paper filter to remove a substance called cafestol, which increases the amount of LDL ("bad") cholesterol in the bloodstream.

If you're not a coffee drinker, you don't need to become one. Knowledge about coffee is evolving, and scientists have found that some people can metabolize (break down) caffeine quickly, while others have a genetic variation that makes caffeine metabolism slower—and that may determine whether coffee has a positive or negative effect on certain aspects of health. For example, caffeine causes the body to lose a bit of calcium, potentially decreasing bone density, but this appears to be more of a concern in those who metabolize caffeine quickly and who drink a lot of coffee. On the other hand, metabolizing caffeine slowly has been linked with an increased risk of high blood pressure and heart disease. If you suspect your blood pressure might fluctuate with your caffeine intake, try gradually cutting back on caffeinated coffee to see if it leads to an improvement in blood pressure. Because people with the genetic variant for slow caffeine metabolism may not notice any symptoms to provide clues that they have the variation, it's a good reason for everyone to stick to moderate intake. Or switch to decaf, which has all the potential health benefits of regular coffee, without the potential downsides of the caffeine.

If you primarily think of tea as a soothing beverage, you may be surprised by everything it has to offer. Black, green, white, and oolong tea all come from the leaves of the same plant, *Camellia sinensis*. This plant is rich in flavonoids, which have antioxidant and anti-inflammatory properties and help relax blood vessels.

About one-third of the weight of a tea leaf is flavonoids, according to Jeffrey Blumberg, PhD, former director of Tufts' HNRCA Antioxidant Research Laboratory. In his view, drinking a cup of tea is like adding a serving of flavonoid-rich fruits and vegetables to your diet. There are few flavonoid health boosters in bottled teas and teas that have been sitting in your refrigerator for several days, however. A more healthful, and cost-effective, option is to hot-brew your iced tea at home before diluting it with ice.

Several health benefits have been linked to tea consumption. One analysis found that drinking three cups of tea daily was associated with an 11 percent drop in the risk of heart attacks. Other studies have linked green tea to better blood cholesterol and triglyceride levels. Interestingly, countries with the highest rates of black tea consumption have lower rates of type 2 diabetes. Regular tea drinking also has been linked with a reduced risk of certain cancers and may support better brain function with age.

## Sugar-Sweetened Beverages

On average, sugar-sweetened beverages (SSBs) account for around 50 percent of added sugars that people consume. Regular soda, lemonade, fruit punch, sports drinks, energy drinks, flavored milks, and most (non-diet) iced teas and coffee drinks are all SSBs. These beverages provide empty calories with little-or-no nutritional value.

SSBs have been linked to weight gain, obesity, heart disease, type 2 diabetes, gout, fatty liver, and a host of metabolic risk factors (including elevated triglyceride levels, high blood pressure, and insulin resistance). A study that examined the link between SSB intake and visceral adipose tissue (VAT)—the fat that surrounds organs—reported that the more regularly participants drank SSBs, the more VAT they gained over the six-year study period. VAT has been linked with greater risk of cardiovascular disease, type 2 diabetes, and certain cancers. Subjects who drank at least one SSB per day had a 27 percent greater increase in VAT volume compared with those who didn't drink any SSBs. If sweet drinks are a part of your daily routine, it's important to take steps to cut back.

### SMART SHIFT — Move Away from Sugar-Sweetened Beverages

Sugar-sweetened beverages account for half of all the added sugars in the Western diet. Try these drink ideas to shift away from sweet drinks.

- Water is always the best choice. If plain water doesn't appeal to you, try putting sliced fruit (like oranges, lemons, strawberries, or watermelon), sliced cucumber or ginger root, or mint leaves in the bottom of the pitcher overnight.
- Coffee is rich in many beneficial compounds, including phytochemicals. Stay away from highly sweetened coffee drinks. If you don't like your coffee black, gradually cut back on the amount of sugar you add, or try stevia, a natural, non-caloric sweetener.
- Tea (black, green, white, and oolong) is rich in antioxidant flavonoids, especially when brewed fresh. Bottled teas are often highly sweetened, but herbal teas (like peach, mango, and mint) make flavorful iced teas that don't need sweetening.
- 100% fruit juice counts as a serving of fruit but is generally missing the fiber of whole fruit. Although the sugar in real fruit juice is natural, there is a lot of it, so stick to 8 ounces or less a day to keep your sugar intake down.
- Sparkling water comes in many different forms.
- Mineral water is naturally fizzy and mineral rich.
- Seltzer is plain water that has been carbonated.
- Club soda is like seltzer, but with minerals added.
- Tonic water is a sugar-sweetened beverage (an 8-ounce serving contains more than 20 grams of sugar and about 90 calories).
- Try sparkling waters with a splash of fruit juice to satisfy that soda craving, or buy brands that are already flavored, but without added sweeteners.

Although you could replace SSBs with artificially sweetened beverages (ASBs) to save calories, some studies suggest that the intense sweetness of sugar substitutes may foster a greater preference to eat sweets and increase appetite. Recent research suggests diet-soda drinkers are more prone to indulging in nutrient-poor treats, which is counterproductive to achieving good health. A report published in 2017 concluded that there's a lack of evidence supporting the role of ASBs in preventing weight gain and a similar lack of evidence on any long-term effects, good or bad, that these beverages may have on health. If you choose to drink diet soda to satisfy your sweet tooth or transition away from SSBs, do so in moderation.

## A Word About Alcohol

Drinking a glass of wine with meals is associated with a reduced risk of chronic diseases, including heart disease and type 2 diabetes. The key with alcohol is moderation, because excess alcohol consumption may have several detrimental effects. Typically, people don't eat less food to compensate for the calories in alcoholic beverages, so drinking wine with dinner every evening will add calories to your diet, which can contribute to weight gain. Alcohol also has been linked to an increased risk of certain cancers, and alcohol can interact with some prescription and over-the-counter medications.

Moderate drinking means no more than one drink per day for women and no more than two drinks per day for men. If you don't currently drink alcohol, there's no need to start.

---

### What Counts as a Drink

Women should limit alcohol intake to no more than one drink a day, and men should have no more than two. A standard drink contains approximately 14 grams of alcohol.

- 12 fluid ounces regular beer
- 8 to 9 fluid ounces malt liquor
- 5 fluid ounces wine
- 1.5 fluid ounces 80-proof spirits, such as whiskey, gin, and rum

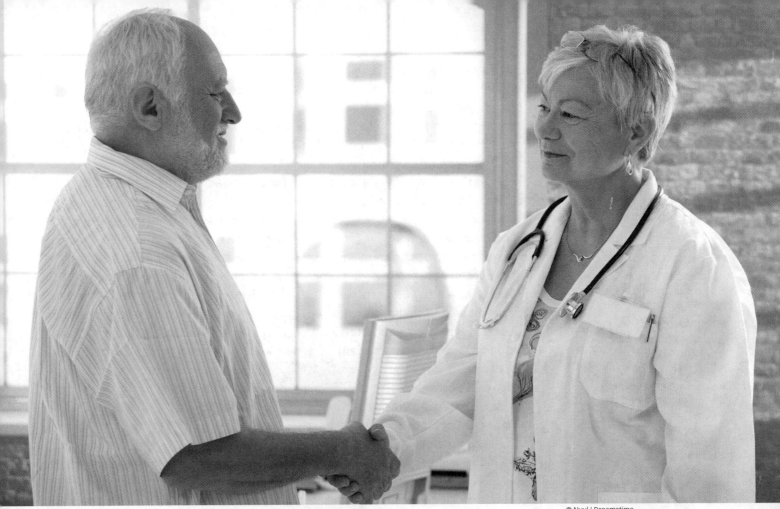

© Nyul | Dreamstime

## 9 Special Health Concerns

If you have special health conditions, like food sensitivities, cardiovascular disease, or diabetes, does standard dietary advice apply to you? Yes and no. It's true that most of the information in this report, as well as in the *Dietary Guidelines for Americans,* is general and geared toward people with no underlying health conditions. However, individuals with special health conditions can still benefit from it. After all, while some general principles of nutrition apply to most people, there's no such thing as a one-size-fits-all diet. This chapter highlights some science-based approaches for adapting basic dietary advice to manage common chronic health conditions. Keep in mind that, if you or someone you care for needs specific guidance on eating to prevent or manage a health condition, you should consult with a registered dietitian nutritionist, your doctor, and other members of your health-care team.

### Food Allergies and Intolerances

If you have a food allergy or intolerance, reading dietary advice that tells you to eat foods you know you need to avoid can be frustrating. But, with a little help, most people can work around food limitations to create a healthful diet. If you're concerned about your dietary pattern, ask for a referral to a registered dietitian nutritionist who can help you build an eating plan that fits your lifestyle and dietary needs.

Food allergies cause immediate, systemic problems, like hives, wheezing, and vomiting, possibly followed later by gastrointestinal symptoms and allergy symptoms like runny nose, coughing, and watery eyes. Food intolerances don't typically cause symptoms immediately after eating, and they're generally localized to your gut (pain, bloating, diarrhea, or constipation),

Your diet can be an important part of managing or preventing common chronic health conditions.

although headaches and skin problems are possible. Sometimes people with an intolerance (or sensitivity) can eat a certain amount of the offending food or food component, but if they pass that tipping point, symptoms arise. Some common intolerances that impact dietary intake are gluten sensitivity and lactose intolerance.

### Celiac Disease

Celiac disease is an autoimmune disorder that can happen in people who are genetically predisposed to it. When someone has celiac disease, ingesting gluten, a protein found in wheat, rye, and barley that makes dough stretchy, leads to damage in the small intestine. The only known treatment for celiac disease is a strict, lifelong gluten-free diet. Giving up every crumb of gluten is essential for the estimated 1 percent of the population with celiac disease. This includes avoiding cross-contamination from bread crumbs in toasters, butter dishes, and cooking utensils and pans, as well as avoiding gluten in medications and supplements. If you have been diagnosed with celiac disease, the basic dietary advice presented in this report does not change, but you do need to choose your whole grains and grain-based foods wisely.

An increasing number of tasty, gluten-free options are available in supermarkets and restaurants, including pizza, cookies, and packaged snacks. Although these options make life simpler, an overreliance on gluten-free goodies could lead eating habits astray. Not only do these processed foods often contain ingredients with little nutritional value, they also can displace healthful, naturally gluten-free foods, such as fruits, vegetables, legumes, nuts, lean meat, fish, poultry, and minimally processed, gluten-free whole grains, including teff, quinoa, and brown rice. If you're newly diagnosed, ask your doctor for a referral to a registered dietitian nutritionist who is knowledgeable about gluten-free diets. Because symptoms of celiac disease may range from "silent" to mild to severe, and

may not include the gastrointestinal tract, it's important that anyone who suspects they can't tolerate gluten be tested for celiac disease while they are still consuming gluten, to get an accurate test result.

### Non-Celiac Gluten Sensitivity

Some individuals may test negative for celiac disease or a wheat allergy but have celiac-like symptoms when they consume gluten. These individuals may be diagnosed with non-celiac gluten sensitivity (NCGS). The dietary remedy is the same as for celiac disease—a gluten-free diet. It's uncertain how many people NCGS affects but available estimates range from 0.6 to 6 percent of the population. Currently, there is no publicly available medical test that can reliably detect NCGS.

### FODMAPs

In some cases, poor tolerance of wheat, rye, and barley products may not be due to celiac or NCGS but, rather, to bacterial fermentation of certain short-chain carbohydrates found in these grains. Other foods that contain various types of fermentable carbohydrates include milk products, fruits, certain vegetables, and legumes. Called FODMAPs (which stands for Fermentable Oligosaccharides, Disaccharides, Monosaccharides And Polyols), these natural sugars and fibers can cause digestive problems in certain people and are being investigated as a potential trigger for irritable bowel syndrome (IBS). When FODMAPs move to the large intestine, they are fermented by bacteria, resulting in production of gas, which may be accompanied by abdominal bloating and pain, as well as nausea, diarrhea, and/or constipation.

Even people who have trouble with FODMAPs can generally tolerate some amounts of these foods. The trick is to find out how much of what foods work best for you. For example, the fruit sugar fructose is a FODMAP, but many people can tolerate a certain amount of fruit at each meal without symptoms; however, since bread made

## FODMAPs

| FODMAP | COMMON FOOD SOURCES | LOWER-FODMAP CHOICES |
|---|---|---|
| Fructans | Wheat and wheat products, rye, barley | Gluten-free bread and pasta; oats, rice, quinoa, teff, and other gluten-free grains |
| | Onion, garlic, artichoke, asparagus, beets, broccoli, Brussels sprouts, cabbage | Green onion tops, chives, garlic-infused olive oil, fresh herbs, green beans, bok choy, bell pepper, carrot, zucchini |
| Fructose | Apples, pears, mangoes, nectarines, peaches, plums, watermelon | Banana, blueberry, kiwi fruit, grapes, melon (except watermelon), orange, pineapple, raspberry, strawberry |
| | Agave nectar (table sugar, honey, maple syrup, and other sugars have about half the fructose of agave) | Artificial sweeteners (tolerance may vary), stevia |
| Galactans | Legumes (beans, peas, lentils, soybeans, peanuts), most soymilk | Meats, fish, chicken, tofu, tempeh |
| Lactose | Dairy (cow's milk, yogurt, soft cheese, cream, custard, ice cream) | Lactose-free milks and yogurt, hard cheese and non-dairy "milks" like almond, rice, and hemp; lactase enzyme pills |
| Polyols | Apples, apricots, avocados, blackberries, cherries, nectarines, peaches, pears, plums, watermelon | Banana, blueberry, kiwi fruit, grapes, melon (except watermelon), orange, pineapple, raspberry, and strawberry |
| | Cauliflower, mushrooms | Alfalfa, bean sprouts, bell pepper, less than 1 cup broccoli, bok choy, carrot, cucumber, green beans, lettuce, tomato, zucchini |
| | Sugar alcohols: Mannitol, sorbitol, xylitol | Artificial sweeteners (tolerance may vary) |

Do not attempt a low-FODMAP diet without the guidance of an experienced physician or registered dietitian nutritionist. Source: Monash University; https://www.monashfodmap.com/about-fodmap-and-ibs/high-and-low-fodmap-foods/

from wheat flour contains other FODMAPs (fructans), having both fruit and a roll could hypothetically be enough to trigger symptoms. Or perhaps you can enjoy an apple and a sandwich, as long as you hold the onions. Following a low FODMAP diet may reduce IBS symptoms.

While avoiding some FODMAPs, such as high-fructose corn syrup and agave nectar in many foods with added sugar, is advisable for everyone, cutting out foods like high-FODMAP whole grains, fruits, vegetables, and dairy makes it difficult to consume enough fiber and some essential nutrients. Ask for a referral to a registered dietitian nutritionist who is knowledgeable about the low-FODMAP diet. After a few weeks on such a diet, you can reintroduce each type of FODMAP, one at a time, to determine your tolerance. Cutting back on FODMAPs has a significant impact on what foods can be included in your dietary pattern, but with the help of an expert and some trial and error, it's possible to construct a healthful, balanced eating plan.

## Lactose Intolerance

Lactose is the naturally occurring sugar in dairy foods. All infants are born with the ability to make the enzyme lactase, which breaks down the milk-sugar lactose. But many adults, especially those from cultures where dairy products are not a diet staple, don't produce enough lactase to adequately break down milk sugar. Lactose intolerance can result in uncomfortable gut symptoms, which typically begin within 30 minutes to two hours of consuming dairy products. Different dairy products have varying amounts of lactose, so the degree of intolerance may differ depending on the dairy product. For some people, simply reducing the portion sizes of milk products or consuming them as part of a meal with other foods can help, while other people may be intolerant even to small amounts. Some people take lactase enzyme pills to help digest dairy products.

Fermented dairy products, such as hard cheeses, yogurt, and kefir, are often better tolerated because the lactose gets broken down during the fermentation process. Another option is to purchase dairy alternatives that are fortified with calcium and vitamin D, such as some soy, rice, almond, and coconut "milks." You can read more about these dairy-free options in Chapter 8. Dairy products are an excellent source of calcium, as well as other important nutrients. If you are unable to consume dairy, make sure you are getting enough calcium from other sources.

## Heart Disease

Along with not smoking and making physical activity a regular part of your life, smart dietary choices are key to protecting your heart health. If you've had a heart attack or stroke or have risk factors for cardiovascular disease like high blood pressure, high cholesterol, or diabetes, you may have been told to change your diet. The good news is, the dietary patterns advocated in the earlier chapters of this book (MyPlate, the DASH diet, and a Mediterranean-style diet) are a move in the right direction.

Research is clear that a heart-smart dietary pattern emphasizes foods that contain specific nutrients known to promote better cardiovascular health—fruits, vegetables, whole grains—in place of refined grains, legumes, nuts and seeds, fish (preferably oily fish, with their healthful omega-3 fatty acids), skinless poultry, and plant-based proteins (such as legumes, soy and quinoa). On the flip side, it's important to limit sugar, sodium, and saturated fat intake and cut trans fat. This means limiting red and processed meats, keeping dairy products low-fat or fat free, and watching for partially hydrogenated oils in processed and fried foods. This type of dietary pattern helps address factors that increase the risk for heart disease, like high blood pressure, elevated cholesterol, diabetes, and obesity.

The following sections will provide more detail on what to emphasize when dealing with specific cardiovascular disease risk factors.

### High Blood Pressure

High blood pressure (or hypertension) is easy to ignore since many people have no symptoms, but it puts you at risk for heart attacks, strokes, and other health issues, so it must be taken seriously. If you have been diagnosed with hypertension, following your doctor's advice and taking any prescribed medication is essential to protecting your health, but there also are steps you can take on your own to help.

To bring down blood pressure, start with a healthful dietary pattern. Then, watch your portion sizes. Blood pressure tends to rise with weight. Basing your meals on reasonable portions of low-sodium,

### Non-Dairy Calcium Sources

The Recommended Daily Allowance for calcium is 1,000 mg for men 19 to 70 years old and women ages 19 to 50 and 1,200 mg for men over 71 and women 51 and older. Milk products are not the only food source of calcium. If you're unable to consume dairy, look to the suggestions below for good calcium sources.*

| FOOD | MEASURE | CALCIUM (MG) |
| --- | --- | --- |
| **Tofu, firm** (prepared with calcium sulfate) | ½ cup | 861 |
| **Almond milk** | 8 fl oz | 451 |
| **Orange juice,** calcium-fortified | 1 cup | 349 |
| **Turnip greens** | 1 cup | 249 |
| **Salmon** | 3 oz | 241 |
| **Black beans** | 1 cup | 239 |
| **Taro** | 1 cup slices | 204 |
| **Spinach** | 1 cup | 194 |
| **Bok Choy** (Chinese cabbage) | 1 cup, shredded | 158 |
| **Currants** | 1 cup | 124 |
| **Herring** | 1 cup | 108 |
| **Tomatoes** | 1 cup | 87 |
| **Peanuts** | 1 cup | 85 |
| **Squash, butternut** | 1 cup cubes | 84 |
| **Edamame** | 1 cup | 72 |

**Supplements:** Growing evidence suggests it may be best to get most of your calcium from foods, rather than supplements, to help guard against excessive intake of calcium and imbalances in bone nutrients. If you need a calcium supplement, look for one that also includes vitamin D, which improves calcium absorption, and magnesium, which is essential for converting vitamin D to its active form in the body. For example, you might choose a supplement that contains 30 to 50 percent of the Daily Value for each of these nutrients to help make up for shortfalls in your diet.

*The amount of calcium that can be absorbed from these foods varies. Source: USDA Food Composition Database

high-potassium foods like fruits, vegetables, whole grains, legumes, and low-fat dairy while upping your activity level will help you reach and maintain a healthy weight. Losing just 5 to 10 percent of your body weight can make a big difference, but good nutrition and regular physical activity alone can improve blood pressure, too.

These suggestions may not be the quick fixes promised by advertisements and websites, but they're proven to work. You can help take control of your blood pressure naturally by changing your diet and lifestyle.

## High Cholesterol

Cholesterol is a waxy, fat-like substance found in all cells of the body. It's essential to the functioning of the human body, where it's used in making hormones, vitamin D, and the bile acids that help you digest food. Cholesterol travels in the bloodstream in small packages called lipoproteins. Low-density lipoproteins (LDL) circulate throughout the body, allowing cholesterol to be deposited in arteries as part of plaque, which can build up, causing hardening, narrowing, and potentially life-threatening blockages. High-density lipoproteins (HDL) remove cholesterol from other parts of your body and bring it to the liver to be metabolized, which lowers the amount of cholesterol in the body. That's why high LDL is considered "bad," and high HDL is "good."

The body can manufacture all the cholesterol it needs, but we also get cholesterol from eating animal products. For a long time, it was thought that consuming dietary cholesterol raised blood levels of LDL cholesterol, but that thinking has recently been called into question. Based on the latest research, the *Dietary Guidelines for Americans* no longer recommends limiting intake of dietary cholesterol to 300 milligrams per day or less. This is a controversial change, and some health professionals disagree.

Most experts do agree, however, that saturated fat raises cholesterol levels and

CVD risk, and that's why this change is not really a big one. Most high-cholesterol foods (like cream, full-fat cheeses, and fatty meats) also contain high levels of saturated fat, so removing the ban on high cholesterol doesn't put these foods back on your healthful plate. Some foods such as eggs, organ meats, and seafood including shrimp and lobster are high in cholesterol but *not* saturated fat, so your doctor or dietitian may give you the go-ahead to enjoy them in moderation.

Soluble fiber helps prevent the digestive tract from absorbing cholesterol, so be sure to choose foods with soluble fiber, like oatmeal, apples, bananas, oranges, pears, prunes, and legumes. Stanols in plant foods also help reduce absorption of cholesterol, which is one of the reasons filling most of your plate with veggies and whole grains and choosing plant-based foods more often can help bring your

### Natural Remedies for High Blood Pressure

While high blood pressure (hypertension) usually has no symptoms, it puts you at risk for heart attacks, strokes, and other health issues. Take medicine as prescribed, aim to lose some weight if necessary, and try these tips to bring blood pressure down naturally.

- **Make a DASH for it.** There's nothing more natural than putting nutritious foods into your body. The plant foods in dietary patterns like the Dietary Approaches to Stop Hypertension (DASH) are naturally low in sodium and high in nutrients (like potassium and magnesium) that help your body regulate your blood pressure.

- **Brew a cup of herbal tea.** If you don't like tea, that's OK. There's no magic elixir that will bring your blood pressure down on its own, but the act of sitting down with a soothing beverage and relaxing can help. Stress can raise your blood pressure, so getting away from it all for a short time every day can help bring your blood pressure down naturally. Going for a walk, taking some deep, calming breaths, meditating, and doing yoga can help, too.

- **Watch your alcohol intake.** Relaxing is good, but don't drink alcohol to relax. Consuming excessive amounts of alcohol can raise blood pressure and interfere with some blood pressure medications. The American Heart Association recommends women consume no more than one alcoholic drink per day and men no more than two.

- **Commune with nature (or the gym).** Getting moving is a natural way to lower your blood pressure. Exercising just 30 minutes a day can help bring your numbers down, so take a walk, hike, jog, swim, or find a fun class or active hobby.

- **Cut the salt.** In the case of high blood pressure, it's not the specific nutrient you eat that helps your health; it's the one you DON'T eat. Too much sodium in your body can lead directly to a rise in blood pressure. Putting the saltshaker down is a start, but you also need to watch out for processed and restaurant dishes, which are often loaded with salt.

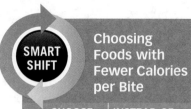
**Choosing Foods with Fewer Calories per Bite**

| CHOOSE... | INSTEAD OF... |
| --- | --- |
| Boiled shrimp | Breaded shrimp |
| Apple | Apple pie |
| Garden salad with light dressing | Macaroni salad |
| Sirloin steak | Barbecue ribs |
| Bran flakes cereal | Granola |
| Skim milk | Whole milk |
| Thin bagel | Bagel |
| Whipped butter | Stick butter |
| Pasta with broccoli | Pasta with cheese |
| Fresh apricot | Dried apricot |
| Grilled, skinless chicken breast | Breaded chicken patty |
| Chocolate-dipped strawberries | Milk chocolate bar |
| Baked potato with salsa | Baked potato with sour cream |
| Angel food cake | Frosted chocolate cake |
| Low-fat popcorn | Potato chips |
| Broth-based vegetable soup | Cream of broccoli soup |

### Mastering Portion Sizes

Don't let packaging and marketing distort your image of how much food you need. Try these tips to manage portions in an oversized world:

- Use 9-inch plates and smaller bowls and serving spoons.

- Don't bring serving dishes to the dining table. Serve food before sitting down.

- Never eat out of a package. Try portioning snacks into individual containers or bags for grab-and-go eating.

- Use a measuring cup occasionally to check how your serving of cereal compares to the package serving size.

- Don't "supersize" it.

- Split restaurant entrees or have half packed up in a to-go container before being brought to the table.

- Order appetizers or small plates as entrees.

- Skip appetizers, creamy-base soup, and dessert when eating at a restaurant.

- Choose nutrient-rich, minimally processed foods, such as whole fruits, non-starchy vegetables, beans, nuts, and low-fat or fat-free yogurt, which are more satisfying than starch- or sugar-rich foods.

blood cholesterol levels down. Replace saturated fat with unsaturated choices, like vegetable oils and fatty fish.

Working to achieve a healthy weight and being as active as your health allows also are important steps that can help lower cholesterol. While you're working on these lifestyle changes, cholesterol-lowering medicines can help lower your heart-disease risk. As your lifestyle changes bring your LDL levels down and HDL levels up, you and your doctor may be able to cut down your cholesterol medications or eliminate them altogether.

## Diabetes

If you are living with type 2 diabetes or have been diagnosed with prediabetes, you may feel that standard dietary advice, which recommends covering three-quarters of your plate with carb-containing plant foods like whole grains and fruit and upping the intake of starchy beans, is not for you. However, the American Diabetes Association now recommends eating a variety of foods, including vegetables, whole grains, fruits, non-fat dairy foods, healthy fats, and lean meats or meat substitutes. Start with a smaller plate (a 9-inch diameter is preferred), fill half of it with non-starchy vegetables, one quarter with whole grains, and one quarter with lean protein. Enjoy a serving of dairy and/or fruit on the side. (Visit the American Diabetes Association's website at diabetes. org for help with meal planning.)

It's also important that you space out your meals throughout the day, don't skip meals, and try not to eat too much food or too much of any one type of food. While highly restrictive diets and carb counting have fallen out of favor for diabetes management, some things remain the same: Learn all you can about diabetes, get physically active, take your prescribed medicine, check your blood glucose as prescribed by your doctor, and go to your appointments. Losing weight, even 10 to 15 pounds, also is very helpful for improving blood-glucose control. To learn more, ask for a referral to a Certified Diabetes Educator or a diabetes education program recognized by the American Diabetes Association.

## Obesity

If you're overweight, even a small amount of weight loss may have big benefits. For example, losing just 5 to 10 percent of your body weight can result in more energy, a better mood, and improved health—although improved nutrition and physical activity habits deserve at least some of that credit. In some studies where participants experienced moderate weight loss of 5 percent or even less, they reported improvements in physical functioning, vitality, and mental health. Modest weight loss also has been found to reduce osteoarthritis knee pain, decrease urinary incontinence, lower the risk of type 2 diabetes, and improve cholesterol and blood pressure levels.

Many different dietary strategies can help you lose weight or prevent weight gain, but the key to success is making changes that you feel good about and can maintain long term. It also is essential that you don't sacrifice the nutritional quality of your diet: A diet plan that excludes or severely limits any one food group or relies heavily on one particular food or food replacement carries the risk of being nutrient-deficient.If you carry extra weight, losing some might be good for your health, but giving your body the nutrients it needs to stay healthy is arguably more important.

The smart shifts recommended throughout this book all are good strategies for reaching or maintaining a weight that's healthy for you, as long as you pay attention to portion control. Numerous studies have found that people tend to base their sense of fullness on the amount or volume of food they eat rather than on how many calories they've consumed. This means that filling your plate with healthful foods like fiber-rich whole grains, water-packed vegetables, and lean proteins can help fill you up and keep you satisfied without excessive calories. Known as "nutrient-dense," foods high in water, fiber, or air have more nutrients per calorie than foods that are lower in water or higher in fat and/or sugar, such as dry snack foods, fatty meats, creamy sauces or dressings, fried foods, and rich desserts. Non-starchy vegetables, broth-based vegetable soups, fruits, low-fat dairy products, air-popped popcorn, and minimally processed whole grains all are examples of foods that pack fewer calories per bite. Nutrient-dense foods can fill many roles in your quest to eat less. A big salad of leafy greens, for example, takes up a lot of space on your plate, requires a lot of chewing, and stretches your stomach, which signals your brain that you've eaten a satisfying amount. Energy-dense foods aren't necessarily off-limits, but be mindful of portion sizes and frequency.

Another helpful technique to help avoid accidentally taking in more calories than your body needs is mindful eating. Slow down and take time to notice the taste, texture, and aroma of your food. This not only can increase enjoyment of the food but also can help you recognize when you're getting full. Avoid eating in front of the computer, while driving, when you're talking on the phone, reading, or watching TV, because you may have no idea how much you're consuming. If you're distracted while you're eating, you're likely to miss your body's signals and overeat. Feelings and emotions such as stress, sorrow, anxiety, and even boredom also may lead you to overeat. Finding ways to address the issues that influence your eating habits is important for physical and mental health and well-being.

## A Word About the Glycemic Index

The glycemic index (GI) is a relative ranking of carbohydrate-containing foods on a scale from 0 to 100 according to how they affect blood sugar levels after eating. This rating scale was initially developed as a food-selection guide for diabetic individuals to improve their glycemic control by classifying foods into low (<55), medium (56-69), and high (>70) GI categories. You might also have heard the terms

**Non-Starchy Vegetables**

- Artichoke
- Asparagus
- Baby corn
- Bamboo shoots
- Beans (green, wax, Italian)
- Bean sprouts
- Beets
- Brussels sprouts
- Broccoli
- Cabbage (green, bok choy, Chinese)
- Carrots
- Cauliflower
- Celery
- Coleslaw (packaged, no dressing)
- Cucumber
- Daikon
- Eggplant
- Greens (collard, kale, mustard, turnip)
- Hearts of palm
- Jicama
- Kohlrabi
- Leeks
- Mushrooms
- Okra
- Onions
- Pea pods
- Peppers
- Radishes
- Rutabaga
- Salad greens (chicory, endive, escarole, lettuce, romaine, spinach, arugula, radicchio, watercress)
- Sprouts
- Squash (summer, crookneck, spaghetti, zucchini)
- Sugar snap peas
- Swiss chard
- Tomato
- Turnips
- Water chestnuts

Source: American Diabetes Association

"slow carbs" and "fast carbs" used. However, use of the GI has gone beyond this original intent and is now being endorsed for use as a labeling tool to guide food choices to reduce chronic disease risk. It also serves as the basis for many popular diets. While there is some clinical data to support a modest benefit of low-GI diets in the management of diabetes, the evidence on the benefits of low-GI diets in non-diabetic populations is mixed, in part because recent research from Tufts University has found that glycemic response to white bread, long considered a high-glycemic food, can vary from person to person, and even in the same person when measured at different times. Rather than getting caught up in numbers, follow a healthy dietary pattern rich in a variety of healthful food choices. When you're choosing vegetables, fruits, whole grains, and legumes, and combining them with adequate protein and healthy fats, you are eating in a way that will promote gentle fluctuations in blood sugar and steadier energy.

☑ CHECKLIST

### Choosing Dietary Supplements

Follow this shopping guide and ask a qualified health professional for further assistance when choosing dietary supplements.

☑ Pick supplements free of unnecessary additives, such as artificial colors (for example, "Red 40") and chemical preservatives (for example, "BHT").

☑ If you see different forms of a vitamin, ask which form is the most active. For example, vitamin D3 is more active than D2 and is generally the better choice.

☑ Pass over multivitamins with synthetic (laboratory-made) vitamin E; "dl-alpha-tocopherol" is synthetic vitamin E, while "d-alpha-tocopherol" is natural vitamin E from food sources and is more potent and better absorbed by the body.

☑ Choose a supplement for your unique needs. For instance, many older adults don't need supplemental iron, which can build up to harmful levels if you get too much.

☑ If you have food allergies or restrictions, such as gluten or soy, check to see if the supplement is free of your allergens. Call the manufacturer of the supplement if you're unsure.

☑ Check for an official mark of purity and quality. Two leading programs are the USP Verified seal and the NSF International seal. Such certifications typically mean the products have been tested and confirmed to contain the ingredients and amounts listed on the package. Get more information about these quality seals and the products that have been tested at usp.org and nsfsport.com.

## Do I Need Supplements?

Sometimes, special conditions make it difficult if not impossible to meet your nutrient needs through foods. That's where appropriate amounts of high-quality supplements can make a difference. Among the most common options are vitamin, mineral, and herbal supplements. Such supplements come in many forms, such as tablets, capsules, powders, and liquids.

In most cases, it's better to get nutrients from food sources—they're absorbed more efficiently and don't have the same safety concerns. Additionally, food components act synergistically to produce beneficial effects, so isolating individual components into supplements could produce unsatisfactory or unexpected results.

If you've made adjustments to your diet and you're still falling short on certain vitamins and minerals, taking a nutritional supplement can help. A multivitamin/mineral supplement that provides around 100 percent of the Daily Value of most nutrients may be adequate for this purpose. However, if your doctor has identified a specific deficiency, you may need to take individual supplements at higher doses, such as for vitamins D or B12, either temporarily or long-term. Here are some examples of groups that may need dietary supplements:

‣ **Older adults.** As you grow older, your calorie needs decline, yet vitamin and mineral needs generally remain the same or, in some cases, increase. Older adults are more likely to fall short on certain nutrients, such as calcium, vitamin D, vitamin B12, and protein. Your doctor can easily test for nutrient deficiencies, such as vitamin D, while other deficiencies aren't as easily detected. See "Nutrients of Concern for Older Adults," in Chapter 2 for a more complete listing of nutrients and top food sources.

‣ **Vegans.** Vegans, and to some extent vegetarians, are at higher risk of falling short on nutrients commonly acquired by consuming animal products, including vitamin B12, vitamin D, calcium, iron, iodine, zinc, and omega-3 fats. For information on food sources of these nutrients, "Nutrients of Concern for Vegans," see Chapter 2.

▶ **Osteoporosis or Lactose Intolerance.** If you can't meet your calcium needs through diet alone, calcium supplements can help. Look for one that also includes vitamin D, which improves calcium absorption, and magnesium, which helps convert vitamin D to its active form in the body. Calcium is best absorbed when taken in doses of 500 milligrams or less. Calcium carbonate should be taken at mealtime to increase absorption. Calcium citrate can be taken with or without a meal.

## Cautions

Unlike medications, which must be proven safe and effective before the FDA allows them to be marketed, dietary supplements do not have to be approved by the FDA or any other agency before they can be sold. It's the responsibility of manufacturers to ensure supplements are safe before they're marketed. Unfortunately, the quality of dietary supplements varies greatly. An investigation by the New York State Attorney General's Office found that over-the-counter herbal supplements often didn't contain the ingredients claimed on the ingredient list. In some cases, the supplements contained unlisted fillers, including wheat and legumes, which are allergens

for some people. Additionally, although you may find various claims about how supplements may help you, many of these products have limited research backing their purported benefits and may not be worth the money.

Some dietary supplements may be harmful when taken in high amounts, for a long time, or in combination with other supplements or certain medications. For example, supplements containing vitamin K, which is involved in blood clotting, interact with anticoagulant drugs, such as warfarin (Coumadin). Other supplements can have undesirable effects before, during, or after surgery. For instance, uncontrollable bleeding is a potential side effect of taking vitamin E, garlic, ginkgo biloba, or ginseng supplements in the two weeks before surgery.

The FDA advises that you consult with a health-care professional before using any dietary supplement, and always tell your surgeon about all supplements you use if you'll be undergoing surgery.

## Final Thoughts

When you have a chronic health condition that affects your food choices, it's natural to focus on foods you should limit or avoid, which can be stressful. However, you'll likely find eating more enjoyable if you shift your attention to what you *can* eat, choosing tasty, healthy foods that can help you manage your disease rather than dwelling on the foods you should pass up.

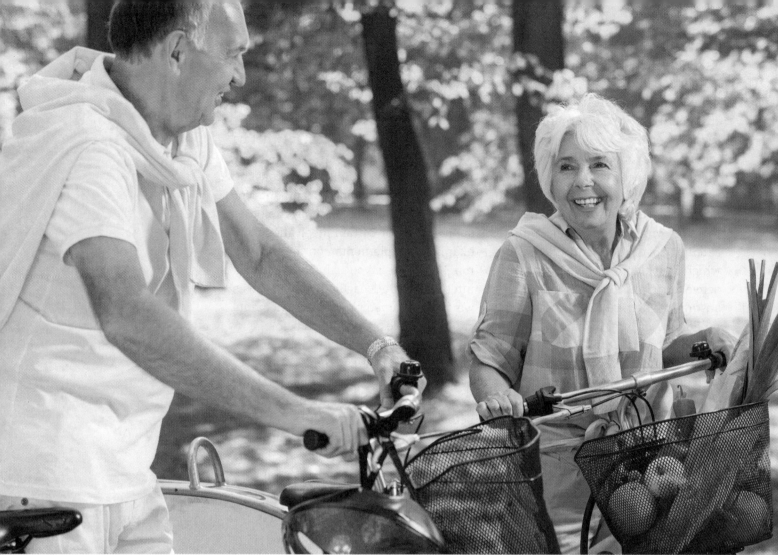
© Katarzyna Bialasiewicz | Dreamstime

A healthy lifestyle can help you preserve the type of life you envision as you age.

# 10 Bringing it Home

Adopting a healthy eating plan that tastes delicious and feels doable for the long term can be a powerful tool to prevent, delay, manage, or even reverse chronic health conditions. That's important to preserve the kind of life you envision for yourself as the years go by, but it's also important for helping to feel energized today. A nutrient-rich diet can help you stay as fit, strong, and independent as possible as you age—isn't that something we all want? Achieving this doesn't require big sweeping changes or an overnight overhaul. Small steps, consistently taken, can really win the race. Without self-judgment, compare where you are now with your diet and lifestyle habits, and where you think you need to be to meet your health goals.

Then decide what small actions you want to start taking today to move in that direction. It's one thing to say you're going to eat more fruits and vegetables, make half your grains whole, include more meatless meals, and reduce salt and added sugars, but it's another to walk your talk. That's especially true when you are navigating all the demands and obstacles of living in the real world. The Tips and Smart Shift features throughout the report are designed to help. This chapter will cover how to prepare foods in ways that won't sabotage your healthy eating goals and how to make restaurant meals fit in your dietary pattern. You also will find a seven-day menu and recipes to inspire your palate and encourage your new dietary goals.

## Shift to Cooking at Home More Often

Home cooking gives you more control over food quality as well as portion sizes. Although many people feel they don't have the time, interest, or skill to make meals from scratch, with a little practice and the right guidance, anyone can put together a fresh, home-cooked meal. No need to try to channel your inner Julia Child.

Cooking is part art and part science. Some people just seem to have a knack for what flavors work well together or when a piece of meat or fish is perfectly done. Others are more comfortable sticking to recipes and using a meat thermometer. The key is finding recipes that meet your dietary goals, are in line with your cooking comfort level, and fit within your timeframe. If you only have 30 minutes to get dinner on the table, or you lack confidence or experience, stay away from complicated recipes. With practice, you'll feel more comfortable in the kitchen. If you're cooking for one or two people, there are many recipe sources that cater to smaller portions, or you can cook in bulk for the week or freeze extra for future meals. There are plenty of resources online and in bookstores to help you do this kind of batch cooking.

Planning is the key to successful home cooking. If you don't have the right ingredients on hand, you're more likely to reach for prepared foods or call for takeout. Choose a few recipes for the week and make a shopping list. Once you've shopped, invest a little time in advance prep. It's easier to throw together a dinner stir-fry or lunch salad if salad greens are washed and vegetables are already cut up and/or portioned. Don't forget to plan for leftovers; if you cook extra protein, you can slice it over salad greens, toss it with whole-grain pasta and sauce, stir it into scrambled eggs, make it into a sandwich, or fold it into tacos or fajitas the next day.

Stock your pantry and fridge with go-to items for quick meals. Cans of beans and diced tomatoes can turn into a quick pasta topping (try adding some olives and frozen or canned veggies), chili (add canned corn and peppers with salsa, chili powder, and other spices), or soup (with canned broth, veggies, and some brown rice or whole-wheat pasta). Make a quick Mediterranean-style salad by mixing a can of tuna with a can of drained white beans and some olives or capers, then dress with a little olive oil and lemon juice and serve over greens.

Stocking up on highly processed convenience foods, such as canned soups and stews, pre-flavored grain and pasta dishes, and frozen meals, may seem like a reasonable way to jump-start home cooking, but these foods typically cost more, are high in sodium, and don't save much time in the long run. Instead of a box of flavored rice, for example, cook a whole grain of your choice in low-sodium chicken broth and add your favorite herbs or spices. For very little effort, you'll have a side dish that's higher in nutrients, lower in sodium, and preservative-free. One smart shortcut is stocking up on frozen vegetables without added sauces—they cook quickly and can be added to any dish to boost your veggie intake.

Using a little olive oil or other healthy plant oil when cooking prevents sticking,

### Planning Menus

Taking a little time to plan your meals in advance will save you time in the long run. Follow these tips:

- **Plan weekly.** Set aside one day a week, such as when the grocery sales flyer comes out, to make a plan of what you'll eat over the next seven days.

- **Consider your schedule.** Think about which days you'll have more or less time to cook, and plan accordingly. Extra servings of homemade soup or casserole stored in your freezer are perfect for busy times.

- **Keep it balanced.** Use MyPlate to guide what you include in your meals. A balanced meal is half vegetables and fruit, one-fourth whole grains, and one-fourth protein-rich foods (ChooseMyPlate.gov).

- **Vary your choices.** Over the course of a week, try to include several different foods from each food group so you get a greater variety of nutrients.

- **Take inventory.** Check your menu against what you have on hand in your pantry and refrigerator. Make a list of what you'll need before you go to the store.

makes dishes more flavorful (fat helps carry flavor across the tongue), and provides heart-healthy fats to help your body absorb fat-soluble nutrients. However, keep cooking fats to a minimum to avoid excessive calories.

Try new flavors or new cooking techniques to expand your repertoire and your palate. Steaming, microwaving, poaching, broiling, and grilling are cooking methods that use less fat, and you can also sauté and stir-fry in a little healthy oil. Roast vegetables to bring out their natural sweetness. Use herbs and spices for flavor to cut back on salt and skip fat- and sodium-laden sauces. Cook meats to the recommended temperature to reduce the risk of food-borne illness.

Find some favorite recipes and keep them in the rotation. On days when you have more time, be adventurous; the more you cook, the easier and more comfortable it becomes. That doesn't mean you'll necessarily grow to love home cooking from scratch, but it will feel easier as you develop the habit, and your body will love the results.

## Tips for Eating Out

Of course, not every meal is eaten at home. Americans consume about one-third of their calories from restaurants and takeout meals. Researchers at Tufts University found that the average meal at a non-chain restaurant had 1,205 calories, similar to meals at chain-restaurants. An average adult needs somewhere around 570 calories per meal (depending on age, activity level, body size, gender, eating frequency, and other factors). Ninety-two percent of the restaurant meals analyzed contained more than 570 calories.

There are many aspects to eating out that get in the way of healthy eating, starting with large portions and what can feel like too many choices. Then there's the fact that many menus lack healthy options, although this is starting to change, as more restaurants offer at least a few

choices that are lower in calories, as well as plant-based and gluten-free options. Browsing a long list of mouth-watering possibilities can make it tricky to stick to smart food choices. Before you go out to eat, put some thought into how you can enjoy your meal while making food choices that support good health.

Many restaurants post their menus online, so you can check their websites beforehand. Also, many chain restaurants and fast-food places provide extensive nutritional information on their menu items. If you must eat on the run, review your options so you'll know what to order ahead of time and avoid being distracted by the glossy images of double cheeseburgers, meatball subs oozing with melted cheese, or Mexican-style fare dripping with sour cream and chipotle sauce.

### Be Mindful of Portion Size

Visualize MyPlate as you consider your meal order. Does the fast-food restaurant offer salad, fruit, or vegetables that can make up half your meal? If the dine-in restaurant offers a bread basket, appetizer, soup, salad, entrée, and dessert, what would all that food look like piled on a single plate? If your fellow diners are willing, ask the waiter not to bring bread to your table. If you're offered free appetizers, politely decline them. Appetizers often are the right size for a meal, so feel free to order one as an entrée. You can even ask to have half the entrée boxed up before it comes to the table or ask for a container at the start of the meal and pack half away for the next day. This can help prevent you from mindlessly eating more than you need to satisfy hunger.

### Make Smart Protein Choices

Protein foods should take up only one-fourth of the space on your plate, but they often dominate restaurant meals. A protein portion, such as a chicken breast, sirloin steak, or salmon fillet, should be about the size (length, width, and thickness) of a deck of cards. Order a smaller option when it's available, or plan to take the excess amount home to enjoy for lunch or dinner the next day.

## Embrace Vegetables and Fruits

If an entrée comes with French fries, ask to swap them out for the vegetable of the day, a garden salad, or any other healthy vegetable option you see on the menu. If there is an upcharge, think of it as money you are investing in your health.

## Build a Better Breakfast

Going to your favorite diner for breakfast? Fruit instead of home fries or hash browns is usually an option. If you order an omelet, request that the cook add mushrooms, onions, peppers, and/or spinach. Skip oversized muffins, which are nutritionally similar to cupcakes, and order whole-wheat toast instead. Avoid the carbohydrate overload trap— pancakes, waffles, toast, biscuits, muffins, and potatoes are all high in carbs. Choose one carb and balance out your breakfast with protein and produce, such as eggs and fruit. If you're going to splurge and order bacon, ask for crispy bacon, which has more of the fat cooked out.

## Consider Preparation Method

Foods that come breaded, battered, smothered, stuffed, or crispy are more likely to be high in saturated fat, and are certainly higher in calories than menu items that have been blackened, broiled, grilled, baked, and steamed.

## Request Condiments on the Side

Avoid drowning your food by asking for salad dressing, barbecue sauce, or gravy on the side. You can dip a forkful of food into the sauce but dipping your fork into the sauce before picking up the food will help you use even less. This will likely cut down on sodium and calories and often reduces saturated fat.

## Drink Wisely

By drinking water instead of soda or alcohol with your meal, you'll save calories and cash. It's common to overlook how many calories beverages can contribute to your diet but including just a few caloric beverages each day can easily add up to more than a quarter of your total calorie needs for the day.

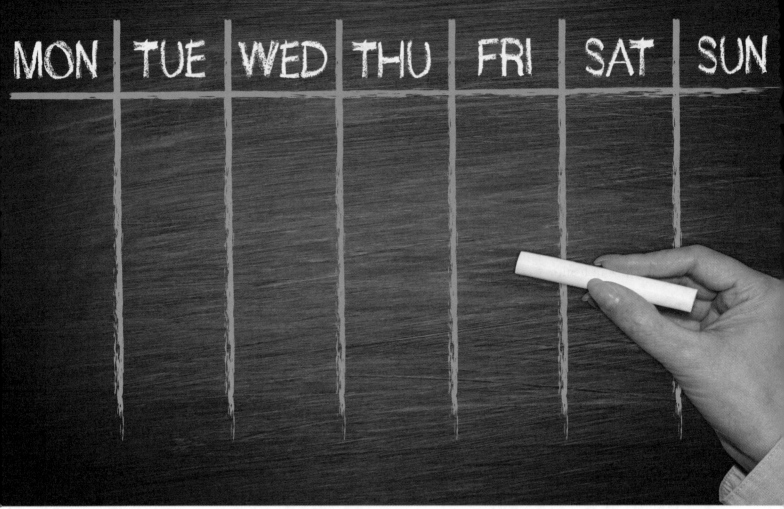

MON | TUE | WED | THU | FRI | SAT | SUN

© Convisum | Dreamstime

Planning a week's menu can help to keep your diet choices healthy and promote your healthy lifestyle.

## 11 Seven-Day Sample Menus

**W**ondering what a healthy dietary pattern looks like in real life? Need some inspiration to get you started? This seven-day menu, based on the principles of the dietary patterns outlined in Chapter 2, is here to help.

These meals are just a guide. The menus in this chapter supply approximately 1,600 calories per day, provided you follow the serving sizes specified. On average, sedentary women age 51 and older need 1,600 calories daily, whereas sedentary men in the same age group need 2,200 calories daily. Your own calorie needs vary because calorie and nutrient needs depend on weight, age, physical activity, health status, lifestyle, and genetic factors. The best gauge of whether you're taking in the right number of calories is to monitor your weight.

If you're following a special diet, the menus can be modified. For example, if you're eating gluten-free, replace a regular English muffin with a gluten-free one. Or, if you're a vegetarian and a stir-fry recipe calls for pork, substitute tofu or beans. If you need more guidance, seek the help of a registered dietitian nutritionist; you can find one in your area by visiting the website for the Academy of Nutrition and Dietetics at eatright.org.

### A Word on Desserts

Shift away from having dessert every day. Pick one or two days per week when you have something special, such as ice cream, cookies, cake, or pie, and keep portion sizes small. Take the time to enjoy your sweet treats by eating them slowly and savoring the taste. If you're counting calories, skip a snack or cut back a bit on meal servings that day. Most days, choose a healthful, fruit-based treat such as the ones listed below.

- Try fruit-based recipes, such as Apple-Raisin Crumble (see recipe section).
- Serve strawberries with a dollop of whipped cream, a drizzle of balsamic vinegar and/or chopped mint.
- Bake apples or pears and sprinkle with cinnamon and a few chopped nuts for crunch
- Grill pineapple slices, peach halves, or plum halves.
- Dip strawberries in low-fat chocolate pudding.
- Freeze grapes, banana slices, or single-serving grapefruit cups (in juice), and then purée until smooth for an easy "sorbet."

Having a piece or cup of fruit is a great way to enjoy something sweet for dessert any day of the week. If you have a "sweet tooth," reach for some fruit when your sugar cravings hit. If you can't shake a chocolate craving, try sitting calmly while a small square of chocolate (preferably dark) melts slowly in your mouth.

## BREAKFAST

- 1 serving Carrot Cake Overnight Oats *(see recipe on page 76)*
- 1 cup nonfat milk
- Black coffee or tea

## Snack

- 1 (5.3-oz) container nonfat plain Greek yogurt with ½ cup fresh or thawed berries (blueberries, strawberries or blackberries)

## LUNCH

- 1 serving Mediterranean Beef and Veggie Wrap *(see recipe on page 79)*

## Snack

- 1 medium apple, sliced and dipped in 1 tablespoon nut or seed butter (peanut, almond, sunflower)

## DINNER

- 1 serving Greek Bean Soup *(see recipe on page 87)*
- Greek Salad: 1 cup romaine lettuce or other salad greens, with chopped cucumbers, tomatoes, ¼ cup crumbled feta cheese, and 1 tablespoon olive oil vinaigrette

DAY 1
DAY 2
DAY 3
DAY 4
DAY 5
DAY 6
DAY 7

## BREAKFAST

- 1 serving Veggie and Cheddar Crustless Quiche *(see recipe on page 77)*
- 1 medium orange
- 1 cup nonfat milk
- Black coffee or tea

## Snack

- 2 rye crisp crackers
- 1 light spreadable cheese wedge

## LUNCH

- 1 serving Greek Bean Soup *(see recipe on page 87)*
- 1 whole-grain roll

## Snack

- ½ cup low-fat cottage cheese with 2 tablespoons raisins

## DINNER

- 1 Walnut Pesto Turkey Burger served on a whole-grain bun with lettuce, tomato, and onion (if desired) *(see recipe on page 88)*
- ½ cup coleslaw with light dressing

## BREAKFAST

- 1 serving leftover Veggie and Cheddar Crustless Quiche *(see recipe on page 77)*
- 1 cup cubed melon
- Black coffee or tea

## Snack

- 1 (5.3-oz) container nonfat plain Greek yogurt with ½ cup fresh or thawed berries (blueberries, blackberries or strawberries)

## LUNCH

- 1½ cup greens topped with 1 Walnut Pesto Turkey Burger *(see recipe on page 88)*

## Snack

- 1 serving Lentil Walnut Spread *(see recipe on page 84)* on 2 rye crisp crackers

## DINNER

- 1 serving Teriyaki Soy Rice Bowl *(see recipe on page 91)*
- 1 cup nonfat milk

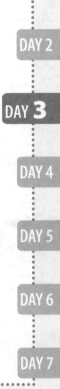

## BREAKFAST

- 1 slice whole-grain toast topped with 1 tablespoon nut or seed butter and ½ medium sliced banana
- 1 cup nonfat milk
- Black coffee or tea

## Snack

- ½ cup cottage cheese
- ½ cup cubed pineapple

## LUNCH

- 1 serving Super Greens Caesar Salad with Roasted Chicken
- 1 whole-grain roll

## Snack

- 1 serving Lentil Walnut Spread spread on bell pepper strips *(see recipe on page 84)*

## DINNER

- 1 serving Spicy Cornmeal-Crusted Alaska Salmon *(see recipe on page 89)*
- ½ cup cooked quinoa
- 1 cup roasted broccoli

## DESSERT

- 1 serving Apple-Raisin Crumble *(see recipe on page 85)*

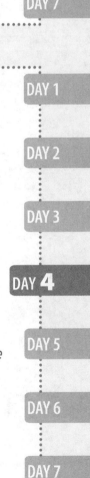

DAY 1

DAY 1

DAY 3

DAY 4

DAY **5**

DAY 6

DAY 7

## BREAKFAST

- 1 slice whole-grain toast topped with spread with ½ an avocado, mashed, and 1 hard-boiled egg, sliced
- Black coffee or tea

## Snack

- 1 (5.3-oz) nonfat plain Greek yogurt with ½ cup fresh or thawed berries (blueberries, blackberries or strawberries)

## LUNCH

- 1 serving Broccoli and Lentil Salad with Turmeric Yogurt Dressing *(see recipe on page 81)*
- 1 lowfat string cheese
- 4 whole-grain crackers

## Snack

- 1 medium apple, sliced and dipped in 1 tablespoon nut or seed butter (peanut, almond, sunflower)

## DINNER

- 1 serving Shrimp with White Wine, Lentils, and Tomatoes *(see recipe on page 90)*
- ½ cup cooked quinoa
- 1 cup chopped, cooked spinach (frozen, fresh or canned), seasoned to taste with lemon juice and black pepper

## DESSERT

- 1 serving Apple-Raisin Crumble *(see recipe on page 85)*

DAY 1

DAY 2

DAY 3

DAY 4

DAY 5

DAY **6**

DAY 7

## BREAKFAST

- 1 serving Blueberry, Apple, and Walnut Baked Oatmeal *(see recipe on page 78)*
- 1 cup nonfat milk
- Black coffee or tea

## Snack

- 2 Pistachio and Apricot Powerballs *(see recipe on page 86)*

## LUNCH

- 1 serving Bulgur Salad with Chickpeas and Herbs *(see recipe on page 82)*
- 15 grapes

## Snack

- ½ cup nonfat plain Greek yogurt with ½ cup fresh or thawed berries (blueberries, strawberries or blackberries)

## DINNER

- 1 serving Alaska Cod Chowder with Black Beans and Corn *(see recipe on page 92)*
- 1 whole-grain roll
- Mixed steamed vegetables with 1 tablespoon vinaigrette

## BREAKFAST

- 1 serving Blueberry, Apple, and Walnut Baked Oatmeal *(see recipe on page 78)*
- 1 (5.3-oz) container nonfat Greek Yogurt
- Black coffee or tea

### Snack

- ¼ cup hummus
- 1 cup raw veggies, such as bell pepper strips, snap peas, cucumber slices, baby carrots, celery sticks)

## LUNCH

- 1 serving Tuna Chickpea Pita Pocket Sandwich *(see recipe on page 83)*
- 1 cup cubed melon

### Snack

- 1 Powerball *(see recipe on page 86)*

## DINNER

- 1 serving Quick Beef Fajitas with Pico de Gallo *(see recipe on page 93)*
- ½ cup brown rice seasoned with lime juice

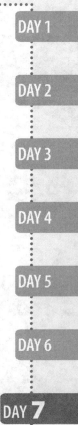

DAY 1
DAY 2
DAY 3
DAY 4
DAY 5
DAY 6
DAY 7

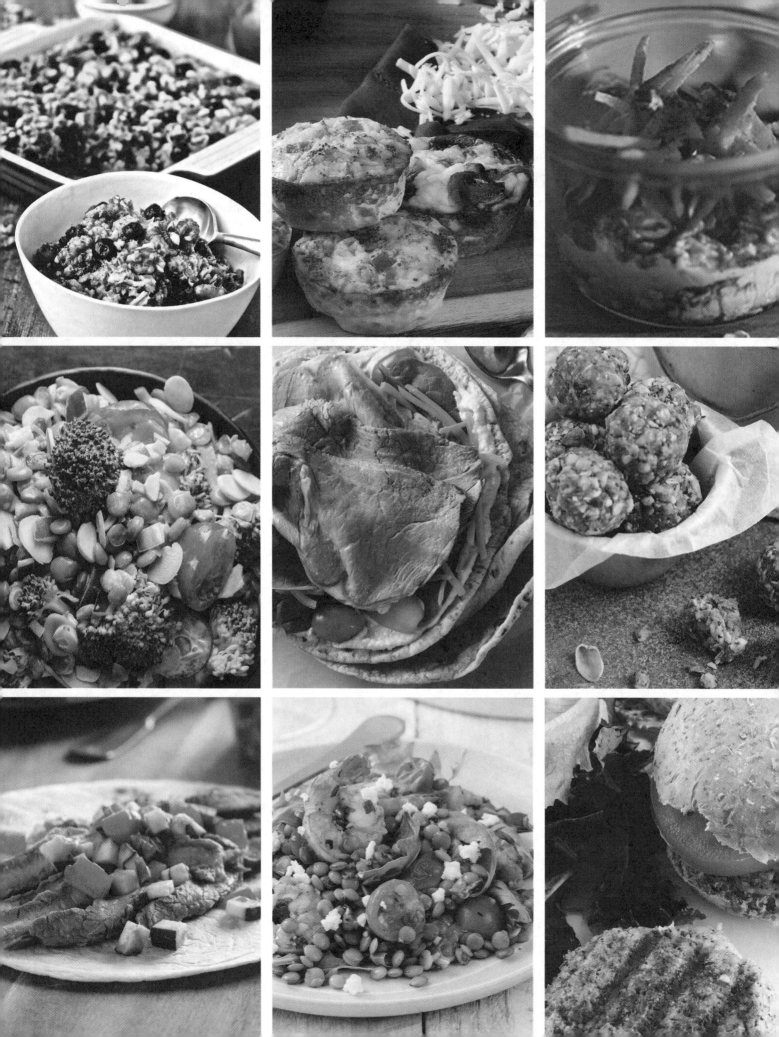

# 12 Recipes

## BREAKFAST

### Carrot Cake Overnight Oats

**Ingredients**

- ½ cup Quaker Oats
- ½ cup nonfat or low-fat milk
- ¼ cup shredded carrot
- 2 tsp maple syrup
- ¼ tsp ground cinnamon
- 2 Tbsp chopped pecans

**Steps**

1. Add oats to your container of choice, pour in milk, and layer carrot, maple syrup, and pecans on top. Sprinkle with cinnamon, place in the refrigerator, and enjoy in the morning.

**Yield:** 1 serving
**Per serving:** 326 calories, 12 g total fat, 1 g sat fat, 11 g protein, 47 g carbs, 17 g sugar, 6 g fiber, 88 mg sodium
**Source:** Recipe courtesy of Quaker Oats

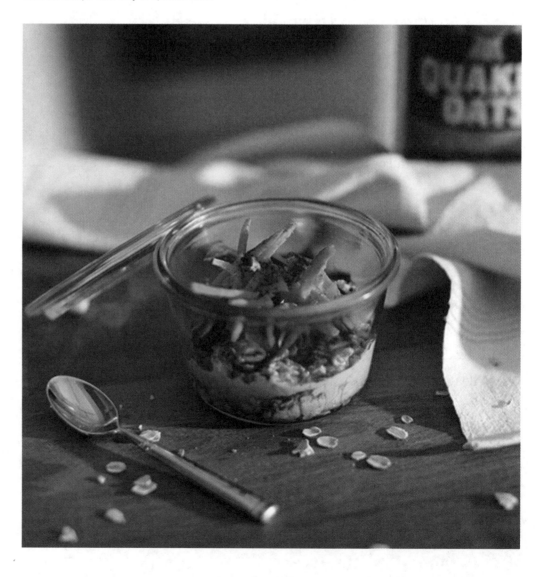

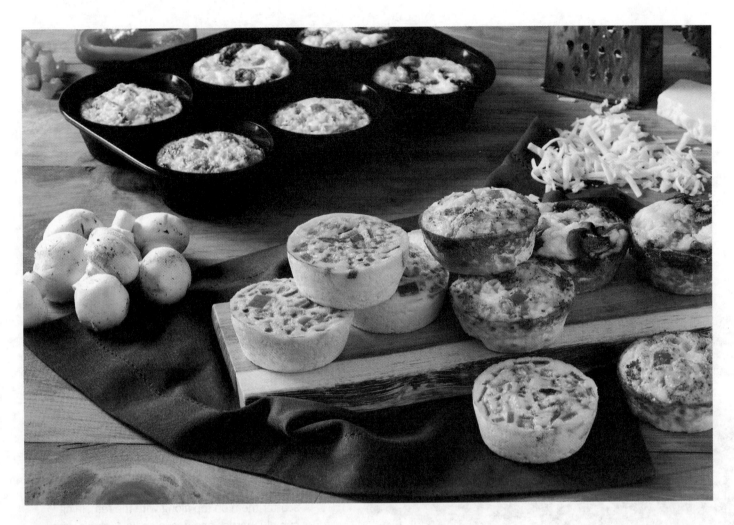

## Veggie and Cheddar Crustless Quiche

### Ingredients

8 eggs

¾ cup 2% milk

¼ tsp each salt and pepper

1½ cups shredded aged Cheddar cheese

1 cup broccoli florets

½ cup finely chopped red onion

½ cup chopped red pepper

### Steps

1. Preheat oven to 350°F

2. Whisk together eggs, milk, salt, and pepper. Stir in cheese, broccoli, onion, and red pepper.

3. Spoon mixture evenly into greased 6-cup jumbo muffin pan.

4. Bake for 35 to 40 minutes or until tops are puffed and knife inserted in center of quiche comes out clean.

5. Run knife around edges of muffin cups; carefully remove quiches.

**Yield:** 6 servings

**Per serving:** 250 calories, 18 g total fat, 9 g sat fat, 18 g protein, 5 g carbs, 3 g sugar, 1 g fiber, 400 mg sodium

**Source:** Recipe and photo courtesy of IncredibleEgg.org

# Blueberry, Apple, and Walnut Baked Oatmeal

## Ingredients

- 1 cup California walnut halves and pieces, divided
- 2 cups old-fashioned rolled oats
- 1 tsp baking powder
- 1 tsp cinnamon plus 1/8 tsp for garnish
- ¼ tsp salt
- 1¼ cups 2% milk
- ½ cup plain low-fat Greek yogurt
- 1 large egg
- ⅓ cup maple syrup
- 2 Tbsp canola or olive oil
- 1 tsp vanilla extract
- 1½ cups blueberries, divided
- 1½ cups finely chopped, peeled apple, divided

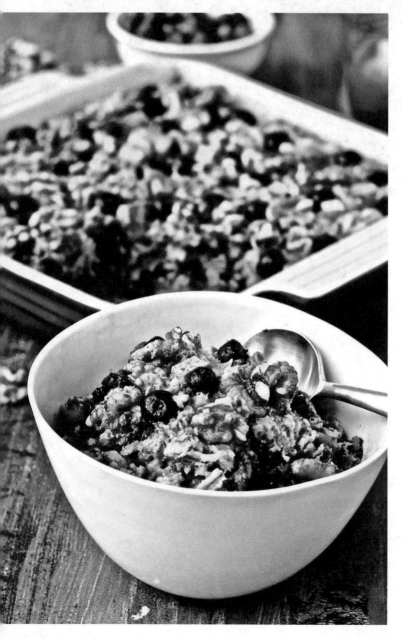

## Steps

1. Preheat oven to 325°F. Spray an 8-inch x 8-inch baking dish with cooking spray. Finely chop ½ cup walnuts and place them in a bowl along with the oats, baking powder, 1 teaspoon cinnamon and salt.

2. Whisk the milk, yogurt, egg, maple syrup, oil, and vanilla together in a large bowl. Add in dry ingredients, 1 cup blueberries and 1 cup apple; stir well. Pour into prepared baking dish.

3. Roughly chop the remaining ½ cup walnuts and scatter them on top along with the remaining ½ cup blueberries and ½ cup apple. Sprinkle with remaining cinnamon.

4. Bake 35 minutes, until the top is golden and the oats are set. Serve warm or at room temperature. Serve as is or topped with milk, Greek yogurt or maple syrup.

**Yield:** 8 servings
**Per serving:** 288 calories, 15 g total fat, 4 g sat fat, 8 g protein, 34 g carbs, 16 g sugar, 4 g fiber, 152 mg sodium
**Source:** Modified recipe and photos courtesy of California Walnuts

# SALADS AND WRAPS

## Mediterranean Beef and Veggie Wraps

### Ingredients

- 3 ounces cooked beef (such as steak, roast, pot roast), thinly sliced
- 1 medium whole wheat flour tortilla (8- to 10-inch diameter)
- Hummus, any variety
- Fresh salad greens
- Additional vegetables, such as:
- Grape tomato halves
- Shredded carrots
- Red bell pepper strips
- Thinly sliced cucumber
- Thinly sliced red onion

### Steps

1. Spread tortilla evenly with hummus, as desired, leaving ¼-inch border around edge.
2. Top with equal amounts salad greens and vegetables, as desired.
3. Top evenly with beef slices. Roll up tightly.
4. Serve with additional greens and veggies as a side salad, if desired.

**Yield:** 1 serving

**Per serving:** 290 calories, 8 g total fat, 2 g sat fat, 22 g protein, 31 g carbs, 2 g sugar, 3 g fiber, 517 mg sodium

**Source:** Recipe and photo courtesy of The Beef Checkoff www.beefitswhatsfordinner.com

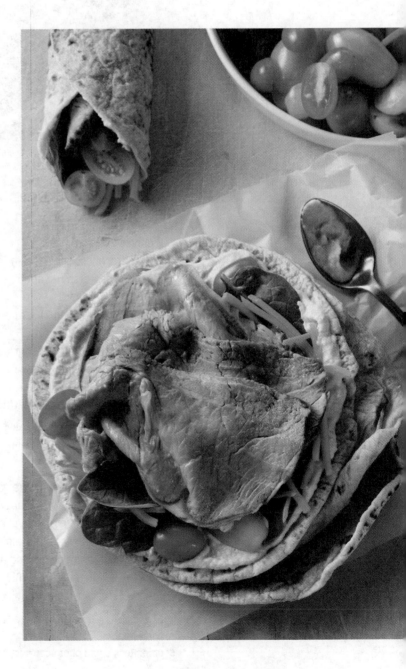

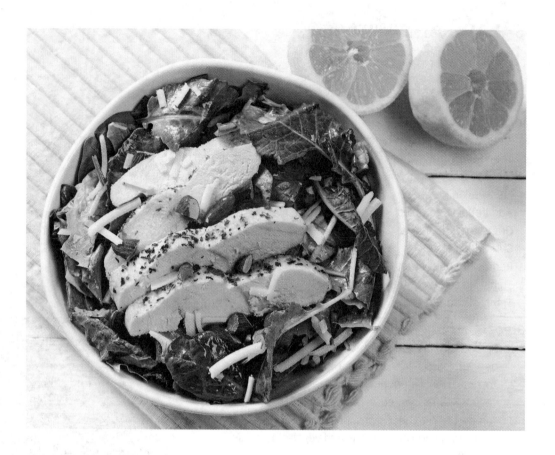

## Super Greens Caesar Salad with Roasted Chicken

### Ingredients

2 cloves garlic, minced

2 Tbsp freshly squeezed lemon juice

1 tsp Worcestershire sauce

1 tsp Dijon mustard

¼ tsp freshly ground black pepper

¼ cup canola oil

3 Tbsp Parmesan cheese, grated, divided

4 cups baby kale leaves

4 cups baby spinach leaves

4 cups chopped romaine lettuce

3 (4 oz) roasted, skinless chicken breasts, sliced

½ cup coarsely chopped toasted almonds

### Steps

1. For the dressing, combine garlic, lemon juice, Worcestershire sauce, Dijon mustard, and pepper in a small glass jar with a lid. Shake well to combine. Add canola oil and 1 Tbsp (15 mL) of the Parmesan cheese and shake well to blend.
2. In large bowl, place kale, spinach, and romaine lettuce and toss well.
3. Drizzle dressing over salad and toss well.
4. Serve salad garnished with sliced chicken and remaining Parmesan cheese.

**Yield:** 6 servings

**Per serving:** 240 calories, 15 g total fat, 2 g sat fat, 22 g protein, 5 g carbs, 1 g sugar, 3 g fiber, 170 mg sodium

**Source:** Recipe and photo courtesy of canolainfo.org

# Broccoli and Lentil Salad with Turmeric Yogurt Dressing

## Ingredients

¼ cup 2% Greek yogurt

¼ cup light mayonnaise

2 tsp whole grain mustard

2 tsp honey

1 tsp white wine vinegar

¼ tsp ground turmeric

Salt and pepper, to taste

SALAD

3 cups broccoli florets (about 1 head of broccoli)

1 cup halved cherry tomatoes

1 cup cooked green lentils

½ cup finely chopped red onion

½ cup sliced, toasted almonds (reserve some for garnish)

## Steps

1. Whisk dressing ingredients together in a small bowl. Season with salt and pepper and reserve.
2. Combine salad ingredients together. Toss dressing with the salad, season with salt and pepper, and garnish with toasted almonds.

**Yield:** 4 servings

**Per serving:** 200 calories, 12 g total fat, 1 g sat fat, 7 g protein, 17 g carbs, 5 g sugar, 5 g fiber, 310 mg sodium

**Source:** Recipe and photos courtesy of lentils.org

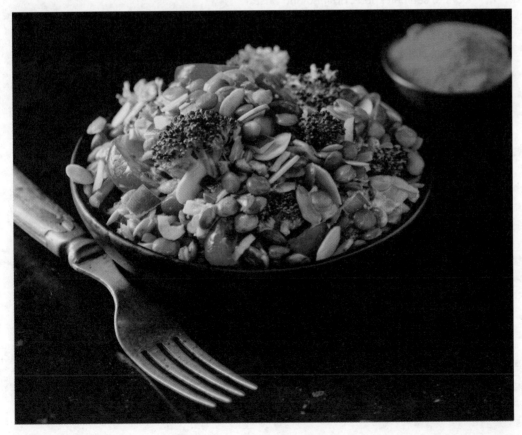

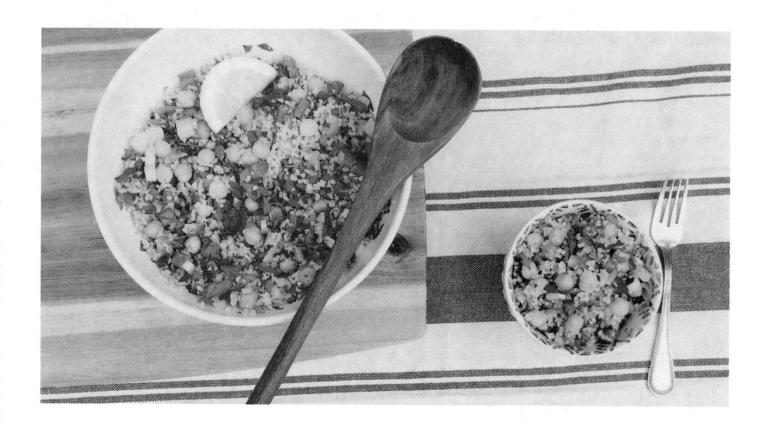

## Bulgur Salad with Chickpeas and Herbs

### Ingredients

1 cup coarse bulgur
1 (15-ounce) can chickpeas, drained and rinsed
2 Tbsp extra virgin olive oil
1 bunch scallions, finely chopped
2 large garlic cloves, minced
¼ cup finely chopped flat-leaf parsley, or a combination of parsley and dill
2 Tbsp finely chopped fresh mint
Juice of 1 lemon
Freshly ground black pepper, to taste

### Steps

1. Prepare bulgur according to package instructions.
2. Heat 1 tablespoon of the olive oil in a large, heavy skillet over medium heat. Add the scallions and cook, stirring, until tender, about 2 to 3 minutes.
3. Stir in the garlic and continue to cook until fragrant, 30 seconds to 1 minute, then remove from heat.
4. In a large bowl, combine the warm garlic and scallion mixture with the cooked bulgur and chickpeas.
5. Add the parsley, mint, lemon juice, and the remaining 1 tablespoon of oil and toss together.
6. Taste and adjust the salt and pepper. Serve hot or at room temperature.

**Yield:** 6 servings
**Per serving:** 230 calories, 7 g total fat, 1.5 g sat fat, 8 g protein, 36 g carbs, 4 g sugar, 8 g fiber, 160 mg sodium
**Source:** Recipe and photo courtesy of Oldways, oldwayspt.org

# Tuna Chickpea Pita Pocket Sandwich

## Ingredients

### DRESSING

⅓ cup fat-free or low-fat Greek yogurt

¼ cup light mayonnaise

2 ½ Tbsp fresh lemon juice

¼ cup chopped fresh parsley

2 tsp chopped fresh or ½ tsp dried crushed rosemary

1 tsp chopped fresh or ¼ tsp dried thyme leaves

### TUNA SALAD

2 cans white albacore tuna (4.5 to 5 oz each) drained well

1 (15-ounce) can chickpeas (aka garbanzo beans), drained and rinsed

¾ cup chopped celery

⅓ cup finely chopped red onion

Salt and freshly ground black pepper, to taste

2 medium tomatoes, sliced

2 cups spinach

2 whole wheat pita pockets

## Steps

1. In a small mixing bowl whisk together Greek yogurt, mayonnaise, lemon juice, parsley, and thyme or rosemary.

2. In a medium mixing bowl add tuna chickpeas, celery, and red onion. Pour Greek yogurt mixture over the top and toss everything to evenly coat. Season with salt and pepper to taste and toss.

3. Slice pita pockets in half then slice through the center to open. Layer in spinach, tomatoes, and tuna salad mixture. Serve immediately.

**Yield:** 4 servings

**Per serving:** 320 calories, 8 g total fat, 1 g sat fat, 28 g protein, 37 g carbs, 9 g sugar, 9 g fiber, 490 mg sodium

**Source:** Recipe and photo courtesy of Jaclyn Bell of CookingClassy.com

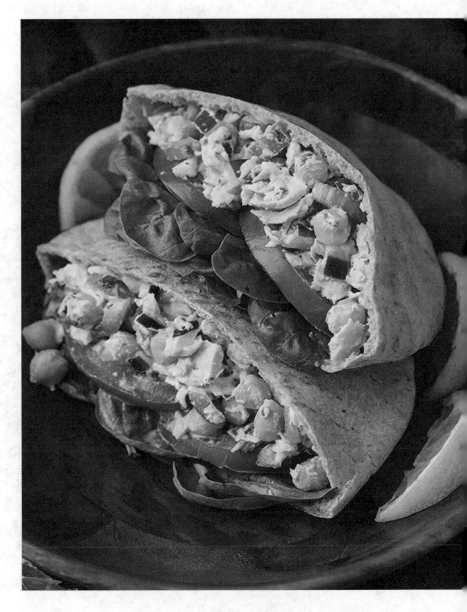

## Lentil Walnut Spread

### Ingredients

- 1 cup lentils, dry
- ½ cup California walnuts, chopped
- 2 tsp Dijon mustard
- 1 Tbsp red wine vinegar
- Salt and pepper to taste

### Steps

1. Wash the lentils, cover with cold water, bring to a boil, and cook until soft, about 1 hour.
2. Drain the lentils and combine with the remaining ingredients in a food processor. Blend until smooth, adding water as necessary to achieve a spreadable consistency.
3. Serve with whole-wheat pita or raw carrots and celery

**Yield:** 8 servings
**Per serving:** 110 calories, 5 g total fat, 0.5 g sat fat, 6 g protein, 11 g carbs, 0 g sugar, 3 g fiber, 30 mg sodium
**Source:** Recipe and photo courtesy of Pulse Canada and California Walnut Commission

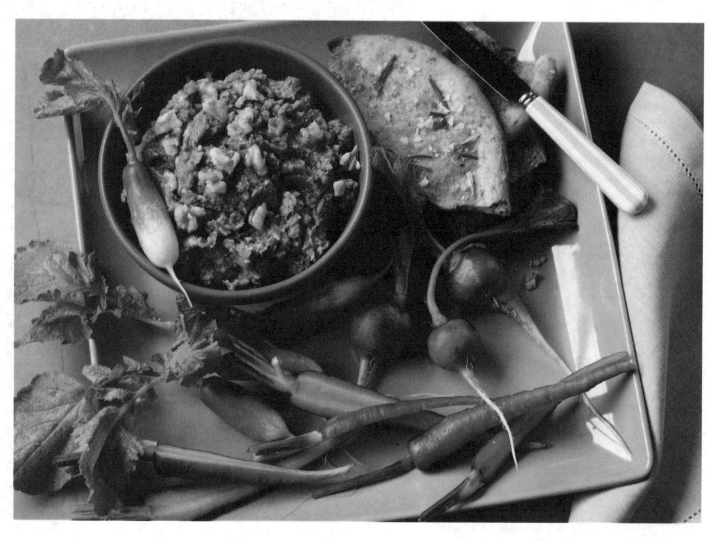

## Apple-Raisin Crumble

### Ingredients

- 8 medium apples (6 McIntosh, Jonathan, or Gala and 2 Granny Smith), unpeeled, chopped into ¾-inch cubes
- ⅓ cup raisins
- 3 Tbsp packed dark brown sugar
- 1 tsp vanilla extract
- 1 Tbsp cornstarch
- 12 gingersnap cookies
- 1 Tbsp canola oil
- ½ tsp ground cinnamon
- 1 Tbsp packed dark brown sugar
- 1 Tbsp maple syrup or honey

### Steps

1. Preheat oven to 350°F.
2. In medium mixing bowl, combine apples, raisins, 2 Tbsp brown sugar (keep remaining 1 Tbsp for step 3), vanilla extract, and cornstarch, toss gently, yet thoroughly until cornstarch is dissolved. Place in an 11-inch x 7-inch baking dish and set aside.
3. Place gingersnaps in small plastic resealable bag. Using back of spoon or meat mallet, crush cookies to coarse texture. Place in small mixing bowl and add remaining ingredients, except syrup. Stir to blend thoroughly and sprinkle evenly over fruit.
4. Bake, uncovered, 45 minutes or until fruit is bubbly. Remove from heat, drizzle syrup evenly over all, and let stand 10 minutes to absorb flavors. Store cooled leftovers covered with plastic wrap in refrigerator up to two days.

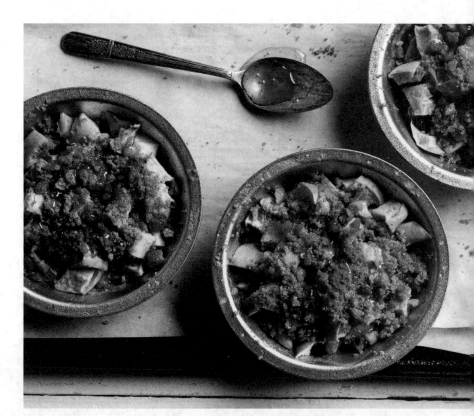

**Tips:** If smaller amount is desired, divide recipe in half and bake in loaf pan as directed.

**Yield:** 8 servings
**Per serving:** 188 calories, 3.5 g total fat, 0.5 g sat fat, 1 g protein, 41 g carbs, 28 g sugar, 4 g fiber, 40 mg sodium
**Source:** Recipe and photo courtesy of canolainfo.org

## Pistachio and Apricot Powerballs

### Ingredients

- ¾ cup shelled unsalted pistachio nuts
- 1 cup ready-to-eat dried apricots
- 2 Tbsp rolled oats
- 1 tsp chia seeds
- 4 tsp peanut or other nut butter

### Steps

1. Put all the ingredients in a blender and blitz until well combined. With wet hands, squash the mixture into balls about the size of a walnut. Store in an airtight container for 4 days.

**Yield:** 10 servings

**Per serving:** 135 calories, 8.5 g total fat, 1.5 g sat fat, 4.5 g protein, 8 g carbs, 5 g sugar, 2 g fiber, trace sodium

**Source:** Recipe and photo courtesy of American Pistachio Growers

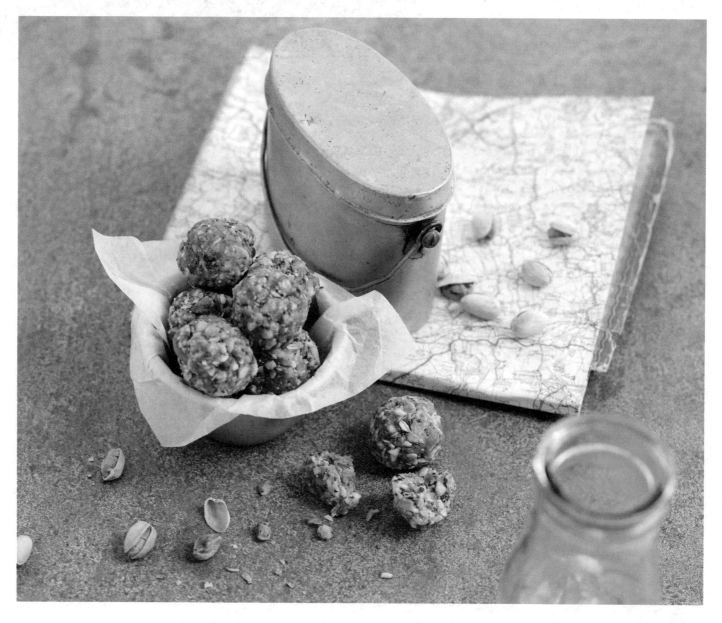

# ENTRÉES

## Greek Bean Soup

### Ingredients

1 lb. dry white beans (cannellini or navy beans)

2 Tbsp extra virgin olive oil

3 to 4 carrots, diced

1 large onion, diced

3 stalks of celery, diced

2 cloves of garlic

1 (14.5-ounce) can diced tomatoes

¼ cup extra virgin olive oil

1 tsp paprika (hot or sweet)

Salt and pepper to taste

### Steps

1. If cooking on a stovetop, you must first soak the beans. Rinse the beans and pour into a large bowl. Cover with 2 inches of water, 1 tablespoon of salt, and let soak on the counter for 4 to 12 hours.

2. In a large pot, starting with a cold bottom surface, sauté the onion, celery, carrots, and garlic in 2 tablespoons of olive oil and add paprika when the vegetables are aromatic.

3. After 2 minutes, add the diced tomato and sauté for 1 minute.

4. Add the soaked beans and cover with enough water to cover the beans by 1 inch and simmer until the beans are tender (30 to 40 minutes).

5. Add ¼ cup of extra virgin olive oil and cook for a few more minutes. The olive oil will make the soup thick and creamy. Add salt to taste.

**Yield:** 8 servings
**Per serving:** 308 calories, 11 g total fat, 2 g sat fat, 14 g protein, 41 g carbs, 11 g fiber, 100 mg sodium
**Source:** Modified recipe courtesy of North American Olive Oil Association

# Walnut Pesto Turkey Burgers

## Ingredients

2 cups fresh basil leaves

¼ cup Italian flat-leaf parsley

2 cloves of garlic

2 cups walnut halves and pieces

½ cup parmesan cheese

1 pound 99% lean ground turkey

1 large egg

## Steps

1. Combine basil, parsley, garlic, walnuts, and cheese in a food processor. Pulse until coarse and just combined.
2. Hand mix with ground turkey and egg.
3. Divide mixture into 8 burgers. Heat olive oil in large nonstick skillet over medium heat. Cook burgers 6 minutes per side or until no longer pink in center.
4. Serve with desired fixings like lettuce, tomato, buns, etc.

**Yield:** 8 servings

**Per serving:** 262 calories, 20 g total fat, 4 g sat fat, 20 g protein, 4 g carbs, 2 g fiber, 122 mg sodium

**Source:** Recipe and photo courtesy of California Walnuts

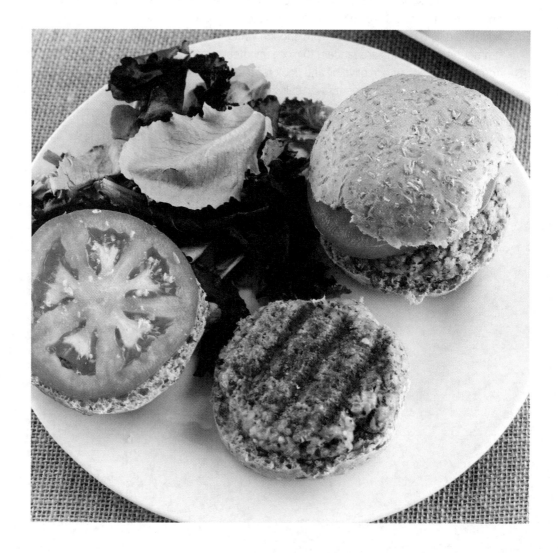

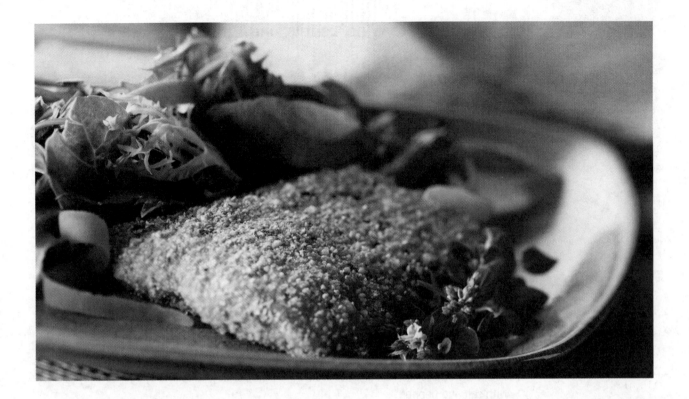

## Spicy Cornmeal-Crusted Alaska Salmon

### Ingredients

⅓ cup medium to coarse-grind cornmeal

1½ to 2 teaspoons favorite spicy seasoning (Cajun, Mexican, Caribbean Jerk, Italian, curry blend, etc.)

½ tsp salt salt

4 skinless Alaska Salmon fillets (4 to 6 oz. each), fresh, thawed, or frozen

1 Tbsp olive, canola, peanut, or grapeseed oil

Nonstick cooking spray

### Steps

1. Blend cornmeal, seasoning, and salt in zip-top plastic bag. Rinse Alaska salmon fillets under cold water, then toss in cornmeal coating.

2. Heat oil in large nonstick skillet to medium-high heat; add fillets to pan. Cook until browned, about 3 minutes. Spray-coat tops of fillets. Turn salmon over gently and cook an additional 4 minutes.

3. If using fresh or thawed fish, check browned fillets for doneness. Cook just until fish is opaque throughout. If using frozen fish, preheat oven to 425°F. Transfer browned fillets to baking sheet and cook an additional 6 to 8 minutes. Cook just until fish is opaque throughout.

**Yield:** 4 servings

**Per serving:** 244 calories, 9 g total fat, 2 g sat fat, 30 g protein, 9 g carbs, 1 g fiber, 432 mg sodium

**Source:** Recipe and photo courtesy of Alaska Seafood Marketing Institute, wildalaskaseafood.com

## Shrimp with White Wine, Lentils, and Tomatoes

### Ingredients

1 pound large shrimp, peeled and deveined

1 Tbsp Herbes de Provence

1½ Tbsp canola oil

⅓ cup dry white wine

2 garlic cloves, minced

1½ cups halved cherry tomatoes

1½ cups cooked whole green lentils

2 cups arugula, kale or spinach

¼ cup chopped parsley

2 Tbsp lemon juice

Salt and pepper to taste

½ cup crumbled Feta cheese

### Steps

1. Rinse the shrimp and pat dry. In a medium bowl, add Herbes de Provence, and shrimp and gently toss until the shrimp are well coated.

2. Heat oil in a large skillet over medium-high heat. Add shrimp in a single layer and cook for 2 minutes. Flip and cook for another minute more, until shrimp are pink and cooked through. Remove to a plate and keep warm.

3. Pour the wine into the skillet and scrape up all of the brown bits. When the liquid is almost reduced, add garlic and cook a couple of minutes, stirring often. Stir in cherry tomatoes and cook for 2 to 3 minutes, until they start to release their juices. Stir in cooked lentils and cook for 2 minutes. Stir in arugula and cook until it begins to wilt.

4. Return shrimp to the pan and stir well. Stir in the parsley and lemon juice. Season to taste with salt and pepper.

TIPS & TRICKS: To make your own Herbes de Provence, stir together: 1 Tbsp each of dried thyme, dried marjoram, and dried basil; 2 tsp dried rosemary, 1 tsp each of dried sage and cracked fennel seeds, and ½ tsp dried lavender (optional). Store in an airtight container.

**Yield:** 6 servings
**Per serving:** 230 calories, 7 g total fat, 2 g sat fat, 19 g protein, 17 g carbs, 6 g fiber, 860 mg sodium
**Source:** Recipe and photo courtesy of lentils.org

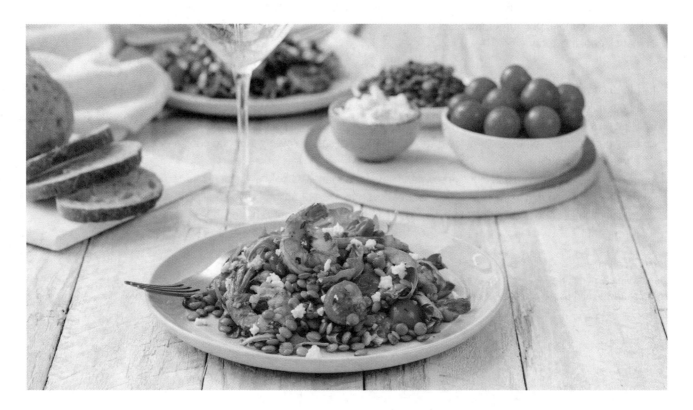

# Teriyaki Soy Rice Bowl

## Ingredients

- 1 Tbsp soybean oil
- 1 14-ounce package firm tofu, cut into ½-inch cubes
- ⅓ cup reduced sodium teriyaki sauce
- ½ cup water
- 1½ cup shredded carrots
- 1 cup frozen edamame, thawed
- 1 cup broccoli florets, cut into ½ inch pieces
- 1 cup red pepper, cut into ½ inch pieces
- 2 cups cooked brown rice

## Steps

1. Heat oil in large frying pan over medium high heat.
2. Add tofu, stirring constantly, for 5 minutes or until lightly browned.
3. Stir in teriyaki sauce, water, carrots, edamame, broccoli, and red bell pepper.
4. Bring to boil and cook, stirring constantly, for 3 minutes or until vegetables are tender and sauce has thickened slightly.
5. Serve over rice.

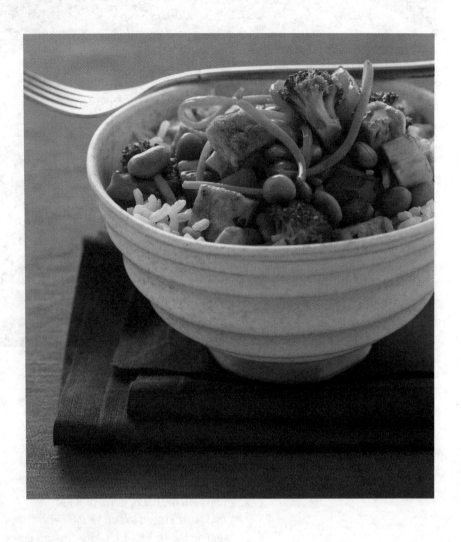

**Yield:** 4 servings
**Per serving:** 450 calories, 13 g total fat, 2 g sat fat, 23 g protein, 64 g carbs, 9 g fiber, 487 mg sodium
**Source:** Recipe and photo courtesy of United Soybean Board, soyconnection.com

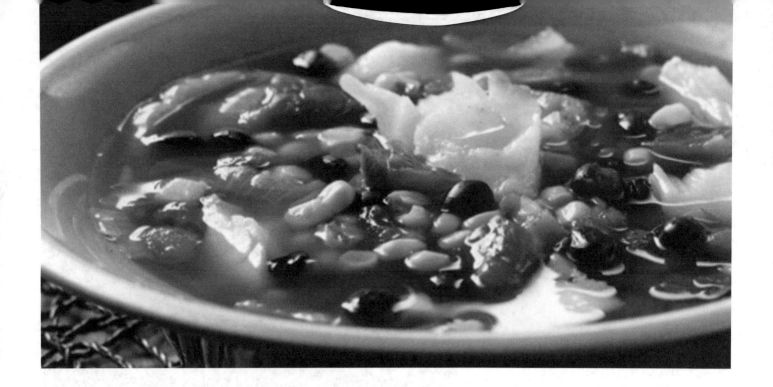

## Alaska Cod Chowder with Black Beans and Corn

### Ingredients

1 medium onion, halved and sliced

1 can (28 oz.) diced tomatoes in juice

2 cans (15 oz. each) black beans, drained and rinsed

2 cans (15 oz. each) corn, drained

1 can (4 oz.) diced green or Jalapeño chiles

½ gallon (64 oz.) fat-free, low-sodium chicken broth

2 Tbsp fresh lime juice

2 tsp chili powder

1 tsp toasted cumin seeds, crushed

½ tsp garlic powder

1¼ pounds Alaska Cod fillets

Tortilla corn chips, if desired

### Steps

1. In large (12-inch) nonstick pan or stockpot, combine onions, tomatoes in juice, black beans, corn, and chiles. Add chicken broth, lime juice, chili powder, cumin seeds, and garlic powder. Bring to boil; reduce to simmer and cook 10 minutes.

2. Rinse any ice glaze from frozen Alaska Cod under cold water. Turn off heat and gently add seafood to sauce, skin side down. Return heat to a simmer. Once simmering, cover pan and cook 4 to 5 minutes for frozen seafood or 2 minutes for fresh/thawed fish. Turn off heat and let seafood rest 5 minutes or until seafood is opaque throughout. Break cooked fillets into chunks, if desired.

3. For each serving, portion soup into shallow bowl and garnish with chips, if desired.

COOK'S TIP: Substitute Alaska Pollock or Sole fillets for Alaska Cod; adjust cook time for smaller fillets if necessary.

**Yield:** 8 servings

**Per serving:** 308 calories, 3 g total fat, 0.3 g sat fat, 29 g protein, 43 g carbs, 11 g fiber, 533 mg sodium

**Source:** Recipe and photo courtesy of Alaska Seafood Marketing Institute, wildalaskaseafood.com

# Quick Beef Fajitas with Pico de Gallo

## Ingredients

1 beef Flank Steak (about 1½ pounds)

12 flour tortillas (6-inch diameter), warmed

## Marinade

2 Tbsp fresh lime juice

2 tsp vegetable oil

2 tsp minced garlic

Pico de Gallo:

½ cup seeded chopped tomato

½ cup diced zucchini

¼ cup chopped fresh cilantro

¼ cup prepared picante sauce or salsa

1 Tbsp fresh lime juice

## Steps

1. Combine marinade ingredients in small bowl. Place beef flank steak and marinade in food-safe plastic bag; turn to coat. Close bag securely and marinate in refrigerator 6 hours or as long as overnight, turning occasionally.

2. Combine Pico de Gallo ingredients in medium bowl.

3. Remove steak; discard marinade. Place steak on grid over medium, ash-covered coals. Grill, covered, 11 to 16 minutes (over medium heat on preheated gas grill, 16 to 21 minutes) for medium rare (145°F) to medium (160°F) doneness, turning occasionally. Carve across the grain into thin slices. Serve in tortillas with Pico de Gallo.

**Yield:** 6 servings

**Per serving:** 452 calories, 18 g total fat, 6 g sat fat, 30 g protein, 39 g carbs, 2 g fiber, 402 mg sodium

**Source:** Recipe courtesy of The Beef Checkoff www.beefitswhatsfordinner.com

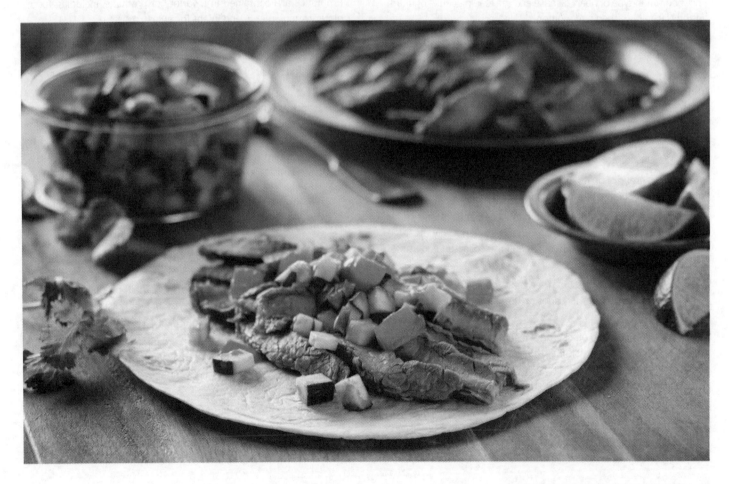

**alpha-linolenic acid (ALA):** An essential fatty acid that belongs to a group of fats called omega-3 fatty acids. ALA is found in plant seeds and oils, such as flaxseed, canola, soy, walnuts, and walnut oils.

**anticoagulants:** Drugs that prevent blood from clotting; these include heparin and warfarin (Coumadin).

**antioxidants:** Substances that experts believe may protect cells from damage caused by unstable molecules known as free radicals, which are produced by the body as a normal byproduct of metabolism. Antioxidants include flavonoids, beta-carotene, lycopene, selenium, and vitamins A, C and E, among others.

**body mass Index (BMI):** A calculation that combines weight and height (weight in pounds / (height in inches x height in inches) x 703. A BMI of 25 to 29.9 is considered overweight, and 30 or higher is considered obese.

**carbohydrates:** Compounds of carbon, hydrogen, and oxygen that form sugars, starches and celluloses, mostly in plants, which provide energy for the body.

**cholesterol:** A waxy, fat-like substance found in foods of animal origin and synthesized by the body. Cholesterol is used for many of the body's processes, including hormone production. Cholesterol can clog arteries if large amounts build up in the blood.

**coronary artery disease (CAD):** A condition caused by the buildup of fatty plaques in the artery walls that narrows the blood vessels and prevents enough oxygen from reaching the heart. CAD is the most common type of heart disease and the leading cause of death in the U.S. in both men and women.

**docosahexaenoic acid (DHA):** A type of omega-3 fatty acid found in fish and algae that is essential for heart and brain health.

**eicosapentaenoic acid (EPA):** One of the two omega-3 polyunsaturated fatty acids (along with DHA) found in fish and associated with reduced risk of heart disease, stroke, improved symptoms of arthritis, and decreased symptoms of depression.

**fats:** Compounds containing fatty acids, which may be monounsaturated, polyunsaturated, or saturated.

**flavonoids:** A group of phytochemicals found in fruits, vegetables, and other plants that act as disease fighters; one subgroup is flavanols.

**gut microbiota:** The complex community of bacteria and other microorganisms that live in the digestive tract, especially the large intestine or colon. The gut microbiome is the collected genome of these microorganisms.

**high-density lipoprotein (HDL):** The "good" cholesterol that carries "bad" (LDL) cholesterol from tissues to the liver, which then removes it from the body.

**hypertension:** High blood pressure. Known as "the silent killer," hypertension is an important risk factor for stroke and heart attack as well as other disorders.

**low-density lipoprotein (LDL):** The "bad" cholesterol that contributes to arteriosclerosis ("hardening of the arteries").

**lipids:** Fats or fat-like substances. Lipid levels in the bloodstream are commonly measured to evaluate cardiovascular health risks. Lipids include LDL cholesterol, HDL cholesterol, and triglycerides.

**monounsaturated fat:** A type of healthy fat in which only one carbon atom is not bound to hydrogen (this also is called a "double bond"). Monounsaturated fats, found in olive, avocado, canola, and other vegetable oils, are generally liquid at room temperature.

**omega-3 fatty acids:** Unsaturated fats found in fish, walnuts, flax-seeds, and some other plant foods that are associated with disease prevention. Diets rich in omega-3s have been linked with a reduced risk of cardiovascular disease and depression, as well as improved brain function.

**omega-6 fatty acids:** A type of unsaturated fat found in many nuts, seeds, and vegetable oils, and in some poultry, seafood, and vegetables. One omega-6 fatty acid, linoleic acid, is essential to the body and is absorbed from our diet.

**phytochemicals (also called phytonutrients):** Compounds in plants that provide flavor, aroma, and color, and protect the plant from microbes and environmental damage. When consumed by humans, phytochemicals are believed to promote health and prevent disease. Many phytochemicals are antioxidants.

**polyunsaturated fat:** A type of healthy fat in which more than one carbon atom is not bound to hydrogen; polyunsaturated fats found in soybean, corn, sunflower, and other vegetable oils are generally liquid at room temperature.

**probiotics:** Probiotics are live microorganisms that, when administered in adequate amounts, confer a health benefit on the host. Probiotics are contained in a variety of products, including foods, dietary supplements and infant formulas.

**protein:** An essential component of all living cells. Dietary protein supplies the body with essential amino acids needed for formation, growth, and repair of cells and tissues in muscles, bones, blood, and skin, as well as the production of enzymes and hormones.

**saturated fat:** A type of fat in which all carbon atoms are bound to hydrogen. Eating a diet high in saturated fat can increase unhealthy cholesterol levels and raise the risk of heart disease. Saturated fatty acids are found primarily in animal foods, especially processed meats, red meats, and full-fat dairy products, including butter. They are generally solid at room temperature. Saturated fat also is found in a few plant foods, such as coconut, palm, and palm kernel oils.

**trans fat:** Fats produced during the partial hydrogenation of vegetable oils, a process that changes polyunsaturated fatty acids from a liquid to a semi-soft or solid state. Trans fatty acids also are found naturally in small amounts in foods from ruminant animals (e.g., cattle and sheep). Relatively small amounts of industrially produced trans fatty acids in the diet can increase the risk of heart disease.

**triglycerides:** A form of fat found in food, fat tissue, and the bloodstream; calories you consume that are not used immediately by the body's tissues are converted to triglycerides and transported to fat cells to be stored. Elevated triglycerides in the bloodstream are a risk factor for heart disease.

**unsaturated fat:** A type of fatty acid that lowers cholesterol levels and reduces the risk for coronary artery disease when it is consumed in place of saturated and trans fats. Monounsaturated and polyunsaturated fatty acids fall into this category.

**Academy of Nutrition and Dietetics**
eatright.org
800-877-1600
120 S. Riverside Plaza, Suite 2190
Chicago, IL 60606-6995

**Almond Board of California**
almonds.com
209-549-8262
1150 Ninth St., Suite 1500
Modesto, CA 95354

**American Diabetes Association**
diabetes.org
800-342-2383
2451 Crystal Dr., Suite 900
Arlington, VA 22202

**American Egg Board**
incredibleegg.org
847-296-7043
8755 W Higgins Rd., Suite 300
Chicago, IL 60631

**American Heart Association**
heart.org
800-242-8721
7272 Greenville Ave.
Dallas, TX 75231

**American Institute for Cancer Research**
aicr.org
800-843-8114
1560 Wilson Blvd., Suite 1000
Arlington, VA 22209

**American Psychological Association**
APA.org
800-374-2721
750 First St. NE
Washington, DC 20002-4242

**The Beef Checkoff**
beefitswhatsfordinner.com
303-694-0305
9110 East Nichols Ave., Suite 300
Centennial, CO 80112

**Canola Council of Canada**
canolacouncil.org
866-834-4378
400-167 Lombard Ave.
Winnipeg, Manitoba, Can. R3B 0T6

**Centers for Disease Control and Prevention**
cdc.gov
800-232-4636
1600 Clifton Rd.
Atlanta, GA 30329-4027

**Dietary Guidelines for Americans 2015-2020**
health.gov/dietaryguidelines/2015/guidelines/
240-453-8280
Office of Disease Prevention and Health Promotion
U.S. Department of Health and Human Services
1101 Wootton Pkwy., Suite LL100
Rockville, MD 20852

**Foodsafety.gov**
foodsafety.gov
U.S. Department of Health and Human Services
200 Independence Ave., SW
Washington, DC 20201

**International Scientific Association of Probiotics and Prebiotics**
isappscience.org
3230 Arena Blvd., Suite 245-172
Sacramento, CA 95834

**National Heart, Lung, and Blood Institute**
nhlbi.nih.gov
301-592-8573
NHLBI Health Information Center
31 Center Drive, Bldg 31
Bethesda, MD 20892

**National Institutes of Health**
nih.gov
301-496-4000
9000 Rockville Pike
Bethesda, MD 20892

**Oldways Whole Grains Council**
wholegrainscouncil.org
oldwayspt.org
617-421-5500
266 Beacon St., Suite 1
Boston, MA 02116

*The Pescetarian Plan: The Vegetarian +*
*Seafood Way to Lose Weight and Love*
*Your Food*
Janis Jibrin, MS, RD; Sidra Forman
Book from Random House Publishing Group, 2014

**Produce for Better Health Foundation**
Pbhfoundation.org
fruitsandveggiesmorematters.org
302-235-2329
8816 Manchester Rd., PMB 408
Brentwood, MO 63144-2602

**Pulse Canada**
pulsecanada.com
204-925-4455
920-220 Portage Ave.
Winnipeg, Manitoba, Can. R3C 0A5

**Tufts' MyPlate for Older Adults**
hnrca.tufts.edu/myplate

**United Soybean Board**
soyconnection.com
800-989-8721
16305 Swingley Ridge Rd., Suite 150
Chesterfield, MO 63017

**U.S. Food and Drug Administration**
fda.gov
888-463-6332
10903 New Hampshire Ave.
Silver Spring, MD 20993

**U.S. Highbush Blueberry Council**
blueberrycouncil.org
916-983-0111
1847 Iron Point Rd., Suite 100
Folsom, CA 95630

**U.S. Pharmacopeial Convention (USP)**
usp.org
301-881-0666
12601 Twinbrook Parkway
Rockville, MD 20852-1790

**USDA Center for Nutrition Policy**
**and Promotion**
cnpp.usda.gov
ChooseMyPlate.gov
202-720-2791
3101 Park Center Dr. 10th Fl.
Alexandria, VA 22302-1594